Pocket Book of
Clinical Neurology

Pocket Book of
Clinical Neurology

By
Richard Suchenwirth

With 86 figures, including 69 diagrams by
Dieter Freiherr Von Andrian

Translated and Adapted by
E. H. Burrows, M.D. and
E. Peter Bosch, M.D.

SECOND EDITION

YEAR BOOK MEDICAL PUBLISHERS, INC.
CHICAGO • LONDON

Author:
Professor Richard Suchenwirth
D3501 Ahnatal/Kassel
Amalienthaler Strasse 35
Federal Republic of Germany

Authorized English translation of the original German edition
published by Gustav Fisher Verlag, Stuttgart, Germany.
Original title: Taschenbuch der klinischen Neurologie, 2.,
erweiterte und verbesserte Auflage

Translator:

E. H. Burrows, M.D.
Department of Neuroradiology
Wessex Neurological Centre
Southampton General Hospital
Southampton, England

Adaptor:

E. Peter Bosch, M.D.
Assistant Professor of Neurology
University of Iowa College of Medicine
Iowa City, Iowa, U.S.A.

Library of Congress Catalog Card Number: 76-20149

International Standard Book Number: 0-8151-8600-2

To My Neurology Students

Preface

Planned to assist the clinician in his handling of neurologic cases, this concise work covers those principles and facts which, in the author's experience, are most frequently required in practice. Wherever possible, reduplication and unimportant or unproved details are omitted. The numerous illustrations are an integral part of the text. A selection of tables for convenient reference will be found at the back of the book.

Separation of the textual matter into topographic neurology and neurologic nosology is retained as far as possible, and no attempt is made to deal with examination technique. The diagnosis becomes obvious at the conclusion of each exercise, but no account is taken of its implications, which would demand a complete review of the patient's somatic, psychologic and sociomedical background. In the orchestra of modern medicine, the neurologist plays only one instrument, albeit an important one.

Investigative techniques receive only brief mention. In many instances, they are unavoidable but they can be overused: the case history, the health of the patient's family and the clinical examination at the bedside are the three pillars of diagnosis and treatment of neurologic diseases. They also form the basis for evaluating progress.

Drugs also receive sparse attention. The reason is that, apart from those that are proved and established, many remain of limited value in modern neurology.

The author thanks his teachers, colleagues and medical students, whose questions always provoke cleared explanations of problems. Credit is also due the publisher for the attractive format of the book.

Here and there, the experienced may criticize passages as being too elementary or too brief, and the author welcomes critical suggestions.

Richard Suchenwirth

Contents

Topographic Neurology 1
Manifestation of Peripheral Nerve, Spinal
     Cord Disorders and CSF Syndromes 3
Cerebral Manifestations 25
Neurologic Nosology 51
Myopathies 55
Diseases of Cranial and Peripheral Nerves 67
Spinal Cord Diseases 101
Cerebellar and Brain Stem Lesions 121
Diseases of the Cerebral Circulation 137
Inflammatory Diseases of the Brain 147
Craniocerebral Trauma 161
Brain Tumors 167
Cerebral Atrophy 179
Epilepsy and Other Seizure Disorders 181
Headache, Facial Pain 187
Appendix 192
References 207
Index 208

Topographic Neurology

The infinitely variable and multifaceted structure of the nervous system ensures that the mode of presentation of neurologic diseases is determined in two ways:

1. The clinical features depend on the part of the nervous system that is affected. Detailed analysis of the function deficit enables us to determine where the disease process is located. Thus, we reach a *topographic diagnosis.*

2. The inherent pattern of each illness is determined by the nature of the disease process, i.e., the cause. The *nosologic (etiologic) diagnosis* indicates whether an infectious (which organism?), vascular, metabolic, degenerative or traumatic cause is responsible for the functional deficit or abnormal signs.

The topographic diagnosis sometimes may permit compelling conclusions about the etiology. More often, after determining the location of the disease process, a painstaking search must be undertaken to discover its cause.

The following criteria lead one to a topographic diagnosis:

a. A careful *case history* obtained by an experienced neurologist. What symptoms and signs did the patient himself observe; when and in what order did they appear? To these questions, the personality of the patient is highly relevant: is he a good observer, does he exaggerate and is he unreliable?

   In patients with seizures, personality changes and behavioral disturbances are additional clues which should be obtained from family members.

b. A systematically performed clinical *neurologic examination.* The physician should never restrict his physical examination at the first encounter to specific parts of the body. Not infrequently unexpected findings in unexpected locations contribute significantly to the diagnosis. (See p. 48, scheme for neurological examination.)

c. *Ancillary investigations* appropriate to the particular clinical problem.

d. *Previous medical records* must be obtained.

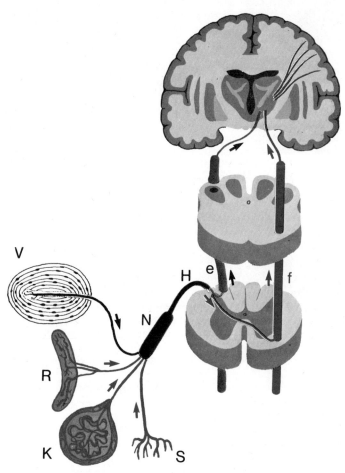

Fig. 1.—Sensory impulses pass toward the brain along the peripheral nerve *(N)* and the posterior nerve root *(H)* into the spinal cord. The impulses arise in the sensory receptors for tactile sensation (Pacinian corpuscles, *V*), heat (Ruffini's corpuscles, *R*), cold (End Bulbs of Krause corpuscles, *K*) and from pain receptors *(S)*, which are distributed widely in the skin. Tactile sensations pass in the posterior *(e)* and lateral *(f)* columns, pain and temperature sensations only in the lateral columns, to the brain.

Manifestations of Peripheral Nerve, Spinal Cord Disorders, and CSF Syndromes

SENSORY DISTURBANCES

The patient describes the symptoms of *spontaneous sensory phenomena* (pain and paresthesias: itching, prickling, burning, sensation of pins and needles, and *sensory deficits* (reduced or absent sensitivity to touch, pain, hot and cold). Spontaneous phenomena of sensation point to a mild dysfunction, a deficit to a more severe disturbance of the sensory system. *Local changes* in the epidermis or subcutaneous tissues may stimulate or damage some of the 500,000 pressure receptors, 3 million pain receptors or 100,000 hot and 60,000 cold receptors, just like a skin disease. The topographic extent of the sensory disturbance will indicate whether the deficit involves only one *peripheral nerve* (most frequently the ulnar nerve, then the peroneal, radial and median) or several nerves (polyneuropathy). All modalities of sensation will be affected within the territory of one or more nerves (cutaneous fields of peripheral nerves, see p. 184). In *diseases of a posterior root* (or the posterior horn cells in certain spinal cord diseases), a segmental loss of all sensory modalities occurs in the corresponding dermatome (commonly S1, L5 and C8). If several segments are involved, a plexus lesion may be present (brachial or lumbosacral). In a transverse lesion causing *damage to the spinal cord* (transverse myelopathy), all sensation below the level of the lesion is lost, including the awareness of bladder and rectal distention.

If the damage is confined to the *anterior spinal cord* (usually syringomyelia), intraspinal tumors and the anterior spinal artery syndrome), a *dissociated sensory loss* may be present: the modalities of pain and temperature are abolished or significantly reduced below the level of the lesion.

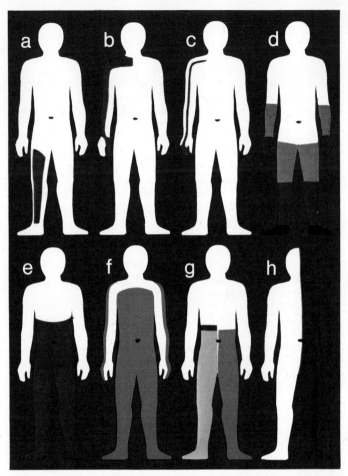

Fig. 2.—Depending on the site of the lesion, all sensory modalities are disturbed (brown), only temperature and pain (red) or only touch (gray). The following types may be distinguished: mononueropathy (e.g., femoral nerve: **a**), plexopathy (e.g., upper brachial plexus **b**), radiculopathy (C7:**c**), distal polyneuropathy **d**), transverse myelopathy **e**), anterior spinal cord syndrome **f**), or unilateral spinal cord syndrome **g**), as well as cerebral hemihypesthesia **h**).

4

Touch sensation is also mediated by the posterior columns; therefore, in such lesions, it escapes extinction.

Unilateral damage to the spinal cord (Brown-Séquard type) is characterized by loss of homolateral tactile sensation (also motor strength) and of contralateral pain and temperature sensation below the level of the lesions. The damaged half of the cord contains the uncrossed tracts for tactile sensation and the crossed pathway for pain and temperature. Ataxia on the side of the lesion is an additional feature, caused by damage to the spinocerebellar tracts. At the level of cord injury, all modalities of segmental sensation are disturbed, since the fibers mediating pain and temperature are affected before they cross. Signs of a segmental deficit of anterior horn cell function are also present; the tendon reflexes are lost at this level.

Thalamic lesions affect all modalities of sensation on the opposite side of the body, causing either irritation or loss; one speaks of a hemihypesthesia or hemianesthesia. At the level of the thalamus, all the tracts subserving sensation have crossed. The sensory phenomena characteristically do not extend to the midline, possess a burning and radiating quality and often are accompanied by excessive affective responses.

Central disturbances that localize to the cerebral cortex (postcentral region) often accompany curtailment of higher perceptive functions (agnosia). Pain perception is affected less severely. Specific features of integrated *epicritic function* are affected early and recover late. They include graphesthesia—recognition of numbers drawn on the skin; pallesthesia—vibration sense (tuning fork); tactile localization; two-point discrimination.

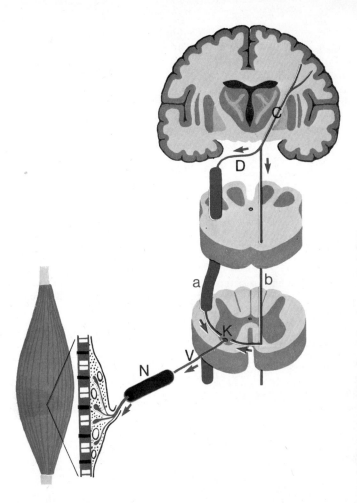

Fig. 3.—Fibers of the pyramidal tract arise in the Betz cells of Area 4 of the cerebral cortex. Most fibers cross and descend in the lateral corticospinal tract *(a)* (to supply the extremity muscles); some uncrossed fibers descend in the ipsilateral anterior cortico-spinal tract *(b)* (to supply the spinal muscles). Motor unit: the anterior horn cell *(K)* innervates the muscle fibers via the anterior nerve root *(V)*, peripheral nerve *(N)* and motor end-plate.

Motor Disturbances

Irritative phenomena may be observed as visible muscular twitches (fasciculations), or with the aid of electromyography, as fibrillations. EMG signs always—and visible fasciculations frequently—are evidence of a lesion of the anterior horn cell or anterior nerve root. Continuous undulations (myokymia) are a less characteristic feature. Sudden contractions of the entire muscle (myoclonic movements) may emanate from a brain stem lesion; complex involuntary movements—often provoked by simple stimuli—are encountered in those diseases of the spinal cord in which pyramidal tract damage has resulted in spinal automatism, which substitutes for central control. In myotonic disorders (muscle membrane irritability due to decreased chloride conductance), percussion of a single muscle belly will result in a persistent contraction lasting for ten seconds or more.

Signs of motor deficit consist of muscle weakness (paresis) or total paralysis. Useful in follow-up evaluation is the grading of individual muscles according to strength: the range extends from 0 = paralysis to 5 = full strength even after prolonged physical activity. Classification of the paralysis depends on the location of the lesion: *myopathies* have a proximal distribution; lesions of the motor endplate (myasthenia) tend to affect the head, neck and bulbar muscles. Here, rapid exhaustion occurs in the presence of initial full strength. In diseases of the *peripheral nerves*, the pattern of involvement follows the anatomic relations; in *nerve root lesions*, the deficit involves a segment (myotome). Transverse spinal cord lesions can cause paraparesis/plegia if only the lower limbs are involved or tetraparesis/plegia if all four limbs are affected. The clinical picture will depend on the level of the lesion in the spinal cord, the former being encountered in thoracic, the latter in cervical cord lesions. Unilateral spinal cord damage causing weakness of one arm or one leg is referred to as monoparesis/plegia. In lesions of the *pyramidal tracts* (containing about 30,000 axis cylinders, with about one million extrapyramidal fibers) the resulting lesion is a hemiparesis/plegia. Different muscle groups may not be affected equally: the forearm, hand and finger extensors, hip flexors, dorsi and plantar flexors of the foot are often totally paralyzed; one speaks of a predilection paralysis (Wernicke-Mann). The more proximal muscles usually are spared.

7

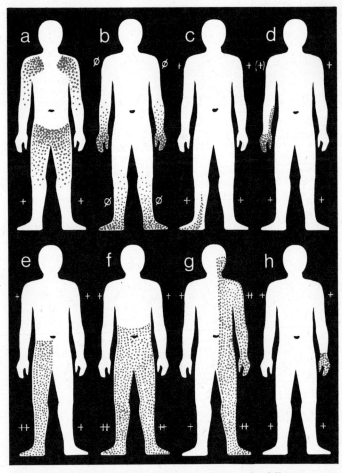

Fig. 4.—Depending on the site of the lesion, the following motor deficits may be differentiated: proximal myopathy (**a**); distal polyneuropathy (**b**); radiculopathy, e.g., L5 (**c**); plexopathy, e.g., lower brachial plexus (**d**); hemisection of the spinal cord (**e**); transverse myelopathy (**f**); contralateral cerebral lesion (**g**); and focal disturbance of the motor cortex (**h**). The degree of the motor deficit may vary from weakness (paresis) to complete paralysis (plegia). Tendon reflexes: absent = $\emptyset$, normal = +, increased = ++.

8

Classification into upper motor and lower motor neuron lesions is important. If only the *upper motor neuron* is involved, the anterior horn and reflex arc remain largely intact but a spastic increase in tone and pyramidal signs develop. If the *lower motor neuron* is damaged, trophic changes will occur in the motor unit of the appropriate segment. The extent and progress of *muscle atrophy* can be gauged by measuring the circumference of muscle bulk in the affected extremity and comparing it with that of the opposite limb. Electrical reactivity of the denervated muscles alters within 3–14 days *(reaction of degeneration)*. Faradic excitability disappears completely. *Rheobase,* as determined with a galvanic current pulse of one second, initially falls and then rises steeply (varies normally from individual to individual and muscle to muscle by 3–8 mA). *Chronaxy,* which is the duration of a pulse twice the rheobasic strength, may rise to levels of 100 msec or more (normal variation always under one msec). The higher the chronaxy the more complete the denervation of muscle fibers. Muscle reactivity also alters qualitatively: in place of the normal situation, i.e., cathodal closure contraction occurring ahead of anodal closure contraction, a reversal or other adjustment may occur. Muscle contractions are prolonged and finally become worm-like. In the most severe neurogenic or anterior horn damage, electrical reactivity ceases completely and the impulse spreads to the adjacent muscles. The prognosis for recovery then is poor. Electromyography reveals fibrillations or positive denervation potentials and a decreased interference pattern (see p. 66).

The motor nerve conduction velocity, which is determined by the latency difference of evoked action potentials between proximal and distal stimulation points on a nerve, is markedly decreased in some peripheral nerve lesions.

The signs of involvement of the lower motor neuron are discussed with the *anterior horn syndrome* (see p. 14).

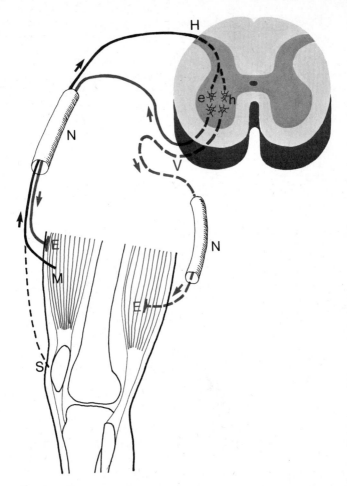

F<small>IG</small>. 5.—The stretch impulse from the muscle spindle *(M)* and tendon receptor *(S)* passes via the peripheral nerve *(N)*, plexus and posterior nerve root *(H)* to the spinal cord. There, it provokes a contraction of the appropriate muscles by stimulating anterior horn cells *(e)* and inhibiting the innervation of antagonist muscles. Invariably the muscle reflex arc is activated in more than one segment.

Reflex Arc, Tendon Reflexes, Muscle Tone

The reflex arc commences in the receptors (muscle spindles, tendons), passes via the peripheral nerve, plexus and posterior nerve root to the posterior horn and then synapses at the anterior horn cells. Here, the second neuron begins: it extends via the anterior nerve root, plexus, peripheral nerve and motor end-plates to the muscle fibers. In healthy subjects, prompt stretching of a muscle (e.g., tendon tapping) provokes a contraction in the muscle that varies in degree; it may be sluggish or lively. This tendon reflex always can be elicited equally on each side. Each muscle possesses a tendon reflex. The following tendon reflexes are easy to elicit and are tested routinely: triceps brachii, brachioradialis, quadriceps femoris (knee jerk) and triceps surae (ankle jerk). Less often, the semimembranosus, semitendinosus, the thigh adductor and tibialis posterior reflexes are tested.

In pyramidal tract injury, loss of inhibitory tone leads to increased reflexes *(hyperreflexia)*. If the reflex arc is damaged in any way, e.g., diseases of the first sensory or lower motor neuron, or of the spinal cord itself at the level of the reflex arc, the reflex is weakened or abolished *(hypo- or areflexia)*.

The same situation applies to muscle tone: in lesions of the upper motor neuron, tone is increased, usually with *spasticity*. Rapid movements prompt severe tonic contractions. If a lesion of the extrapyramidal system is present, *rigidity* may occur also. The increased tone appears as a continuous resistance ("lead-pipe rigidity") or is interrupted by a series of consecutive "gives" in the "cog-wheel rigidity"). If either the afferent or the efferent part of the reflex arc itself is interrupted at the appropriate spinal cord level, tone is diminished or abolished *(hypo- or atonia)*.

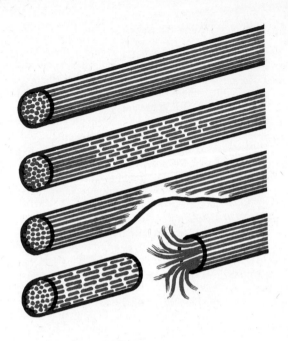

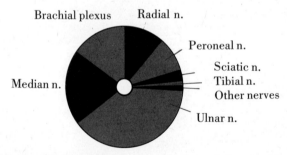

Fig. 6.—Diagrammatic representation of a normal nerve, neurapraxia, axonotmesis and neurotmesis. Circular diagram left: the incidence of peripheral nerve lesions (after Krenkel).

Almost invariably, signs of both sensory and motor involvement are present in peripheral nerve disease. Paresthesias commonly appear first, followed by a disturbance of epicritic sensation and, finally, an impairment of protopathic sensation. Initially, motor weakness (paresis) appears only after prolonged physical activity, later also at rest. If nerve transmission is disturbed or abolished, without interruption of anatomic continuity, the condition is called *neurapraxia*. If the axis cylinder is interrupted but the nerve sheath remains intact, *axonotmesis* is present. In the latter, the functional deficit is complete and anatomic and functional recovery takes considerable longer. The worst prognosis and most severe findings accompany *neurotmesis*, in which the entire nerve is severed. No recovery can occur without surgical treatment (nerve grafting). The regenerative activity in the proximal remnant stimulates numerous axis cylinders to sprout—which, however, lack the guidance of the distal nerve sheath. A club-shaped overgrowth of the proximal stump occurs (neuroma). Neurosurgical repair of the sheath is aimed at approximating the regenerated axonal sprouts to the distal remnant, in order to reestablish a growth pathway to the motor end-plates. In this way, functional recovery is made possible in some cases. Regeneration takes time; it is reckoned to progress at the rate of 1–2 mm a day. All peripheral nerve injuries show sensory disturbances in the central part of the appropriate cutaneous field of innervation, lesser deficits in the boundary zones due to overlapping motor paralysis and later atrophy of the muscles and disturbances of autonomic function, including sweating.

13

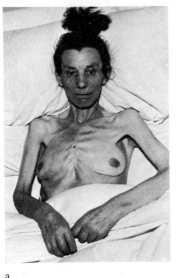

a

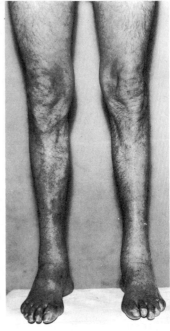

c

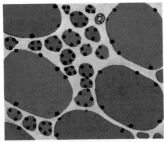

b

Fig. 7.—Muscle wasting in anterior horn cell disease or lower motor neuron involvement. Example: Amyotrophic lateral sclerosis **(a)**. Diagrammatic muscle biopsy: group atrophy of muscle fibers of a motor unit due to disease of the appropriate anterior horn, or its axon. Very large muscle fibers are interspersed with very small ones—not intermediate-sized fibers **(b)**. Muscle atrophy ("stork's legs") in Charcot-Marie-Tooth's disease (peroneal muscular atrophy) **(c)**.

14

If regeneration fails to occur, the muscle tissues undergo structural changes. The affected tendon becomes fixed in a position of contracture and the joint space is obliterated. The deficient muscular activity as well as vasomotor disturbances adversely affect the circulation and lead to inadequate circulatory perfusion: the affected extremity becomes pale, cyanotic and sometimes edematous. After two years, the situation may be regarded as permanent.

If the nerve regenerates per se (in axonotmesis and neurapraxia) or after successful operation, the slow return of function occurs—first motor function and then protopathic sensation—in reverse order to its loss at the time of the injury. Primitive movements again become possible when slight power returns, and functional overlap mediates a return of the sensory modalities of touch and temperature. Functional stimulation by means of graduated exercises leads to a slow rebuilding of the muscle mass and a return of higher motor and sensory function. A significant measure of the extent of peripheral nerve damage is the determination of motor (and also sensory) *nerve conduction*. By electrical stimulation of a nerve along various points and by recording the motor latencies of the evoked muscle action potential on the oscilloscope of an EMG apparatus, one can calculate the conduction velocity of the electrical impulse if the distance between stimulation points is known. Normal values vary from nerve to nerve (about 50–70 m/sec); in neurapraxia, it is slightly lower, in neurotmesis, considerably reduced.

Muscle biopsy will reveal atrophy of the individual fibers belonging to damaged motor units: the fibers are reduced in size and show histochemical abnormality. Regeneration produces large groups of histochemically identical muscle fibers. Only a few motor nerve fibers need survive for this *grouping according to fiber type* to occur.

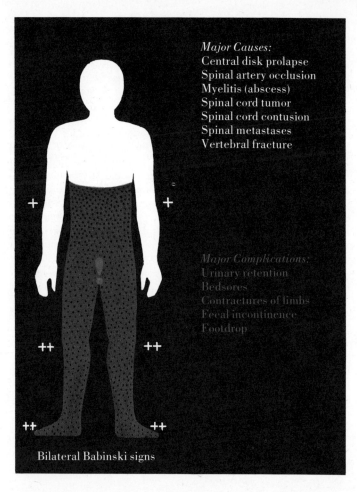

Major Causes:
Central disk prolapse
Spinal artery occlusion
Myelitis (abscess)
Spinal cord tumor
Spinal cord contusion
Spinal metastases
Vertebral fracture

Major Complications:
Urinary retention
Bedsores
Contractures of limbs
Fecal incontinence
Footdrop

+   +

++   ++

++   ++

Bilateral Babinski signs

FIG. 8.—Acute paraplegia has many causes and late complications. The clinical picture is simple: motor deficit (mild weakness to total paraplegia), disturbances of all sensory modalities and double incontinence. If the lesion involves the lower thoracic and lumbar spinal cord, and initially in spinal shock syndrome, the paralysis is flaccid, otherwise spastic with increased muscle tone and positive Babinski signs.

16

A combination of sensory, motor and autonomic as well as *bladder and rectal disturbances* is characteristically present in spinal cord syndromes. The level of spinal cord damage (at which the posterior nerve root lesion produces the sensory changes and the anterior nerve root lesion the motor and autonomic changes) can be differentiated from that produced by damage to the descending and ascending tracts of the spinal cord. *In transverse myelopathy*, the entire cross section of the spinal cord is affected at the level of the lesion. In the corresponding segments there is damage of the lower motor neuron with muscle atrophy and hypotonia, absent reflexes, flaccid paralysis, autonomic dysfunction (pilo-, vaso- and sudomotor dysfunction and, if the lesion involves the conus, bladder and rectal disturbances). All function ceases: below the level of the lesion no sensory modalities can be perceived. The motor system (pyramidal and extrapyramidal tracts) is interrupted. Voluntary movements no longer are possible (or are severely restricted in incomplete lesions).

The spinal cord below the level of the lesion remains anatomically intact. Afferent impulses from the periphery (not appreciated by the patient) and residual efferent impulses (over which the patient has no conscious control) produce a functional situation in which central control is lost: muscle reflexes mediated via the intact arc become accentuated and tone increases (spasticity). Primitive responses *(automatisms)* can be elicited by peripheral stimulation; mass movements may occur. Various abnormal signs now are present: Babinski's, *Trömner's and Rossolimo's* (contraction of the finger or toe flexors on flicking the distal phalanx or after brisk tapping). The skin remains unchanged. Contractures threaten free movements of the elbow, hip and knee joints, and the end result is drawn-up legs with footdrop.

Automatism also affects *bladder and rectal function:* overfilling (of which the patient is not aware) which leads to precipitate emptying ("automatic bladder").

17

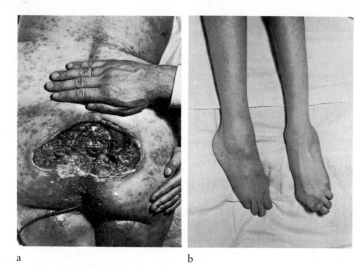

a   b

FIG. 9.—Severe decubitus bedsores, appearing after many
months of recumbency despite all nursing precautions in a patient
with an inoperable spinal cord tumor (a). Footdrop (and spontaneous Babinski signs) in spastic paraplegia (b). These are two major
complications of prolonged paraplegia. Bedsores affect the shoulders, elbows, heels and hips as well as the buttocks. The risk of
sepsis is present constantly.

Sensory stimulation of the extremities provokes involuntary flexion contractions of the legs.

All such automatic movements need not appear immediately after the paraplegia. Inititally, a flaccid paralysis is present, with *urinary and rectal retention* (danger of vesicoureteral reflux with hydronephrosis)—the spinal shock syndrome.

If the spinal cord lesion interrupts the bladder (rectal) reflex arc, all control of bladder (rectal) function is lost. Urine drains away as it collects in the bladder. The detrusor muscle is flaccid. (Ascending urinary tract infection is a real threat due to constant leakage from the bladder).

The patient's permanent recumbency and his inability to carry out physiologic movements, favors the onset of *decubitus ulceration* (bedsores), which may become extensive. The most valuable preventive measures are regular and intensive nursing care of the skin, including turning the patient onto his stomach regularly, and meticulous attention to sterility.

Unilateral spinal cord damage produces the Brown-Séquard syndrome (see also p. 5), with dissociated anesthesia below the level of the lesion; i.e., homolateral tactile and contralateral pain and temperature sensory loss, homolateral pyramidal tract signs and homolateral ataxia. Bladder and rectal disturbances are less frequent. At the level of the cord injury, segmental sensory loss of all sensory modalities and lower motor neuron signs are present.

The *anterior spinal cord syndrome* in syringomyelia and the anterior spinal artery syndrome produce sensory loss (pain and temperature) and pyramidal and extrapyramidal tract dysfunction below the level of the lesion. Involvement of the anterior horn damages the lower motor neuron, causing fasciculations, muscle atrophy, absent reflexes and an abnormal electromyogram.

Conus lesions produce saddle anesthesia, loss of the anal reflex, disturbances of micturition (autonomic bladder) and impotence.

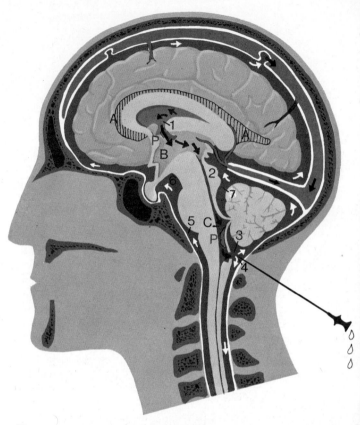

Fig. 10.—Lateral view of the cerebrospinal fluid pathways. Cerebrospinal fluid *(CSF)*, produced in the lateral ventricles *(A)*, passes through the foramen of Monro *(1)*, 3rd ventricle *(B)*, aqueduct of Sylvius *(2)*, 4th ventricle *(C)*, foramens of Magendie and Luschka *(3, 4)*, thence around the brain and spinal cord. The CSF is absorbed via Pacchionian granulations into the superior sagittal sinus. Areas where the subarachnoid space over the surface of the brain is widened are called cisterns, each named according to its particular location. They may be demonstrated by pneumoencephalography.

The cerebrospinal fluid (CSF) volume amounts to about 150 ml in adults. After being produced in the choroid plexus (P), it passes from the lateral ventricles (A), through the 3rd ventricle (B) and 4th ventricle (C) into the central canal of the spinal cord and over the surfaces of the brain and spinal cord (Fig. 10).

Obstruction of the CSF outflow (foramen of Monro (1) between the lateral and 3rd ventricles; Sylvian aqueduct (2); foramina of Luschka and foramen of Magendie; and (3) between the 4th ventricle and cisterna magna (Fig. 10) leads to increased intracranial pressure and mass effects. The result is a hemispheric syndrome (if the obstruction lies at a foramen of Monro) or a *generalized raised intracranial pressure syndrome*, which is especially common in aqueductal occlusions. Focal lesions such as tumors and inflammatory processes producing adhesions may cause obstructive hydrocephalus and obliterate the cerebral cisterns (cisterna magna, pontine, interpeduncular, chiasmatic, lateral [sylvian], interhemispheric, ambient). Atrophic cerebral lesions enlarge these spaces. Information about the nature and extent of these lesions may be obtained by special investigations involving the intrathecal injection of air (pneumoencephalography), radionuclides (radioisotope cisternography) or computed tomography. Lumbar spinal puncture is carried out between the L2–3, 3–4 or 4–5 intervertebral spaces with the patient lying on his side, curled up like a cat. Pressure measurements always should be made; in the relaxed and recumbent patient, values of 100–200 mm water are normal. Higher levels represent raised CSF pressure and values below 50 mm, a low-pressure state, the latter resulting from inadequate CSF production (aliquorrhea). If during lumbar puncture the patient tenses his abdominal muscles, the CSF level in the manometer may quickly rise to double its initial valve and then fall as quickly. Compression of the neck veins also raises the CSF pressure (Queckenstedt's sign); failure of jugular compression to produce a rise indicates an obstruction of the spinal CSF compartment. Before spinal tap, exclude papilledema.

21

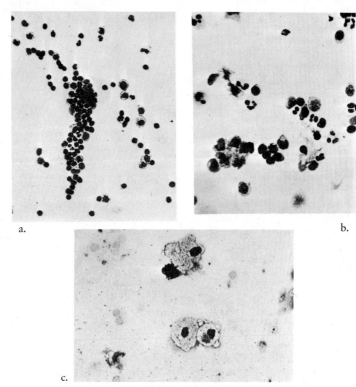

a.

b.

c.

Fɪɢ. 11.—Sayk preparations of CSF cells: **(a)** Lymphocytic meningitis, with scattered monocytes. **(b)** Cerebral abscess: segmented nuclei, monocytes and plasma cells. **(c)** Gitter cells in cerebral degenerative processes.

Typical CSF Picture

	Cell Count	Protein
Normal	1–5	20–35 mg/100ml
Multiple sclerosis	20–100	30–50 mg/100 ml
Neurosyphilis	20–200	60–100 mg/100ml
Spinal tumor	5–20	100–1,000 mg/100 ml
Brain tumor	1–9	30–100 mg/100 ml
Viral meningitis	500–1,500	50–250 mg/100 ml
Purulent meningitis	1,000–60,000	100–1,000 mg/100 ml

22

Disease processes involving the subarachnoid or adjacent spaces produce changes in the composition of the CSF. Normally, the *total protein content* amounts to 20–35 mg/100ml, albumin 60%, alpha and alpha-2 globulins 5%, beta globulin 16% and gamma globulin 8%. The total protein is considerably higher in spinal cord tumors ("total spinal block"), meningitides and brain tumors, less markedly raised in cerebrovascular and atrophic processes and only slightly raised in multiple sclerosis. The globulin content is high in general paresis. In subacute inflammatory lesions, the immunoglobulins are elevated, particulary IgA; in multiple sclerosis, particularly IgG (levels over 7). The IgM level is higher than normal in nondegenerative diseases. A typical feature is a first-zone *colloidal gold* curve, even in the presence of a normal total protein, in *multiple sclerosis* and a left mid-zone curve in florid *general paresis*.

The *glucose level*—the normal value being half that of the blood glucose—is reduced in bacterial meningitis, especially tuberculous meningitis. The *electrolyte values* are not of significant diagnostic interest (chloride slightly higher, potassium and calcium levels definitely reduced, sodium equal to serum).

The *cell count*, as recorded in the 3.2 mm^3 Fuchs-Rosenthal counting chamber, may show important changes; normally there are 1–8 cells, lymphocytes and monocytes. In disseminated encephalomyelitis (multiple sclerosis) and neurosyphilis, the cell count is 15–200, in poliomyelitis 100–1,000, in viral meningitides 500–2,000, in purulent meningitis 2,000–60,000 cells. Using the Sayk sedimentation chamber, polymorphonuclear WBCs are found in acute bacterial infections, eosinophils in *parasitic* diseases, tumor cells (sometimes) in *brain tumors and metastatic lesions*, *erythrocytes* and later *hemosiderin-laden phagocytes* following hemorrhages and lipophages in degenerative processes.

In the Guillain-Barré syndrome (polyneuritis), the cell count is normal and the protein content is markedly increased ("albuminocytologic dissociation"). Usually the cause is a polyradiculitis.

Inspection of the CSF may give certain clues: bloody fluid with xanthoderomic supernatant is associated with subarachnoid hemorrhage, turbid fluid with meningitis, xanthoderomic with markedly increased CSF protein.

23

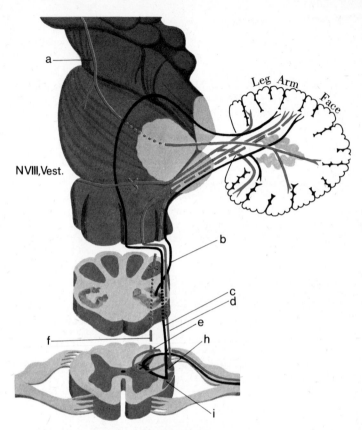

Fig. 12.—Coordination and diadochokinesia are subserved by the neuronal system of the cerebellum and spinocerebellar tracts (*i* and *c:* Gowers' bundle, located ventrally; *h* and *d:* Flechsig's bundle, located dorsally). Afferent inputs reach the cerebellum from the cerebrum *(a)*, the vestibular system *(N VIII)* and the posterior columns *(f)*; efferent pathway via the inferior olivary nucleus modulates the anterior horn cells. Potential disturbances of this neuronal system are legion.

Cerebral Manifestations

INCOORDINATION ATAXIA

Coordination of motor activity is regulated by the cerebellum. It receives afferent input from muscle and joint receptors via the dorsal roots and spinocerebellar tracts and receives and modulates impulses originating in the cerebrum and brainstem, leading to the lower motor neurons, anterior roots, peripheral nerves and muscles. A wide variety of lesions at various levels can result in dysfunction of coordination; e.g., myopathies and polyneuritides.

A pronounced *ataxia* accompanies lesions of the cerebellum and spinocerebellar tracts.

Cerebellar hemisphere lesions produce limb ataxia, with intention tremor, dysmetria, hypermetria, megalographia (large, flowing handwriting), disturbances in maintaining rhythms and in judging the weight of objects. Movements against resistance (rebound phenomenon) cannot be curtailed; for example, if pressure from the examiner's hand is removed suddenly, the patient cannot raise a full glass of water to his lips without spilling it. Speech is poorly articulated and consonants can be spoken only with difficulty: the patient utters explosive, stuttering words. Muscle coordination is defective (dyssynergia), as is the rapid alternating movements of agonist and antagonist muscles (dysdiadochokinesia).

Cerebellar vermis lesions usually cause truncal ataxia: the patient has difficulty in sitting up or walking.

Spinal ataxia produces particularly severe ataxia, since all afferent and efferent pathways are involved. A broad-based gait is present, which, if combined with a loss of muscle tone, gives rise to the so-called lusty legs appearance, as in tabes dorsalis. At an advanced stage, the patient is unable to walk unassisted or to care for himself.

The following illustrate disturbances of coordination: finger-to-nose, heel-knee-shin and finger-touch tests. Examples of the patient's handwriting (megalographia) and figure drawing may also emphasize them.

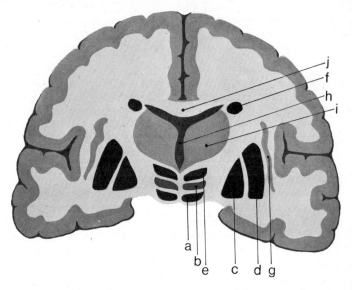

Fig. 13.—Diagrammatic representation of the principal components of the extrapyramidal system: *(a)* substantia nigra; *(b)* red nucleus; *(c)* globus pallidus; *(d)* putamen; *(e)* subthalamic nucleus (corpus Luysii); *(f)* caudate nucleus. Also shown: claustrum *(g)*; 3d ventricle *(h)*; thalamus *(i)*; corpus callosum *(j)*. The clinical deficit depends largely on the location of the disease process.

The *extrapyramidal system* also subserves movement. Disorders of the system produce hyperkinesia (involuntary movements of individual muscles or muscle groups) and/or akinesia (widespread poverty of movement through the absence of associated movements). Rhythmic movements of fingers, hands, feet and head are referred to as *tremor*. In the Parkinsonian syndrome, resting tremor occurs at 4–7-second intervals. The finger movements resemble pill rolling (counting money). This type of tremor—as well as the poverty of movement and rigidity—commonly appears and indicates a lesion of the substantia nigra. The tremor in Wilson's disease affects the shoulder girdle, so-called "wing beating." Both types of tremor increase at rest, disappear during sleep and diminish during volitional movements.

Athetosis is a term applied to slow movements affecting particularly distal parts of the extremities: the fingers are splayed and execute involuntary vermicular movements. The cause is a lesion of the globus pallidus, usually acquired in early life. It may be bilateral (double athetosis). *Chorea* evidences brief, lightening movements affecting more proximal muscle groups. The lesion is chiefly in the corpus striatum (caudate nucleus) and produces its effect by disinhibition of the substantia nigra, reticular substance and the anterior horn.

Hemiballismus, i.e., coarse, flailing movements of one side of the body that cause the patient to fall down, is produced by a lesion in the subthalamic nucleus (corpus Luysii). *Torsion dystonia* denotes repetitive, slow rotatory movements about the vertical axis involving the head, neck and trunk muscles, which usually is caused by a lesion of the putamen. Resistance of the antagonist muscles gives the patient a tormented appearance. *Spastic torticollis* is viewed as a subform, in which the rotatory movements are limited to only the head and neck muscles. *Myoclonus*, i.e., sudden jerking movements of individual muscles, is observed in myoclonic epilepsy.

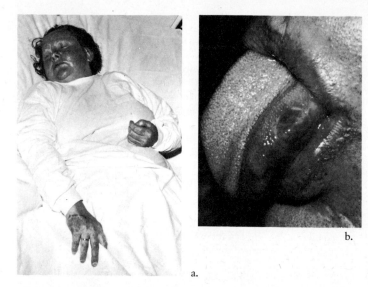

a.

b.

FIG. 14.—(a) Adversive attacks with head deviation to the side of the lesion and rhythmic movements of the contralateral (left) arm, due to a cerebrovascular accident. (b) Scars due to tongue biting in generalized epileptic seizures. Typically, the scars lie on the edge of the tongue, being well demonstrated by adjacent connective tissue scarring. In grand mal attacks, the precise time of onset should be taken into account: morning attacks ("waking attacks") point to symptomatic epilepsy and night attacks ("sleep attacks") to idiopathic epilepsy.

The generalized seizure (grand mal) may have a preceding *aura* (breath of wind), which usually consists of tactile, visual, olfactory or auditory phenomena; even scenic situations are reported. Next follows the *tonic phase*, associated with contraction of the thoracic and laryngeal muscles—often a shrill scream and the patient almost always collapses: his complexion becomes cyanotic and he lapses into unconsciousness. The *clonic phase* consists of rhythmic 1–2-second contractions of all muscles. Injuries may occur: *tongue biting* is common; associated autonomic dysregulation causes over-salivation ("foaming at the mouth"), profuse sweating and incontinence (usually urinary, sometimes fecal (and ejaculation). A period of *clouding of consciousness* follows the clonic phase; usually it lasts a few minutes but the patient may sleep for hours (postictal-sleep). The aura indicates an epileptic focus, and its nature may indicate the location. An olfactory aura ("uncinate fit") points to a focus in the uncal gyrus, a tactile aura to a focus in the postcentral region, visual phenomena to one in the calcarine fissure. Focal attacks can occur in isolation without a generalized seizure ("sensory Jacksonian attack"). A lesion in the precentral region may present clinically as a "motor" *Jacksonian attack* that commences in a single muscle group (often the thumb) and from there the rhythmic contractions spread to affect an entire limb or side of the body ("march of the convulsion"). The march occurs within seconds and may lead to a generalized seizure. Rotation of the head to the side of the focus ("the patient looks at the focus") is typical of *adversive attacks*. Any lateralizing evidence of paroxysmic motor activity should be recorded; it may possess localizing significance. *Infantile spasms* are a type of epileptic attack that occurs in early childhood; later, another variety is seen—a number of minor attacks (petit mal), which may be accompanied by sudden collapse *(myoclonic drop attacks)* or by peculiar mouth movements *(oral petit mal)* or prepubertal fits *(impulsive petit mal)*. The pupils almost invariably fail to react to light during seizures.

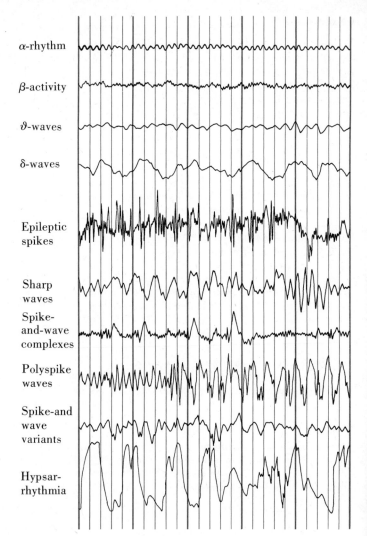

α-rhythm

β-activity

ϑ-waves

δ-waves

Epileptic
spikes

Sharp
waves

Spike-
and-wave
complexes

Polyspike
waves

Spike-and
wave
variants

Hypsar-
rhythmia

Fig. 15.

Electroencephalography (EEG)

The technique of electroencephalography enables potentials that arise from the surface of the brain, amplified many times, to be recorded. Depending on the manner in which the electrodes are placed over the skull, unipolar or bipolar readings may be obtained (unipolar = against a neural electrode applied close to the ear; bipolar = between two points on the head). The variations in potential are recorded as waves, by means of a continuous paper print-out. Comparison of the electrical currents in the various leads provides information about the potentials existing over the surface of various parts of the brain. Healthy adults at rest and with their eyes closed show an alpha-wave pattern of 11 Hz (7.5–13) and an amplitude of up to 50 mV; one speaks of a Berger rhythm (after the father of electroencephalography, Hans Berger). *Beta waves* (14–30 Hz) appear when the subject opens his eyes and α *waves* recede. In neonates, numerous δ *waves* (1–3 Hz) are present, and, later, ϑ *waves* (4–7 Hz) are increasingly prominent. In older children, α *waves* predominate. Brain dysfunction of whatever type leads to an α *suppression* and, scattered bursts of slow waves. The more prominent these bursts the worse the dysfunction. The slow wave pattern over all parts of the brain is referred to as *generalized delta activity* or, if only over a specific part, as a ϑ *or* δ *focus*. The latter finding indicates a focal lesion affecting the cortex at the particular site. Electroencephalography permits no conclusion about the nature of an underlying lesion—it may be tumor, abscess or focal edema surrounding a vascular lesion. Regular β waves are a feature of *barbiturate intoxication*. Epileptiform diseases are characterized by increased activity (convulsive spikes = runs of sharp β activity; consulsive spikes = ϑ activity). They may appear unexpectedly in an otherwise unremarkable recording (bursts), or focally in relation to a circumscribed epileptiform lesion, or in a typical combination: characteristic of *petit mal* epilepsy of childhood is a succession of spikes and waves in 3/second cycles *(spike-and-wave complexes)* or bilateral discharges *("centrencephalic epilepsy")*.

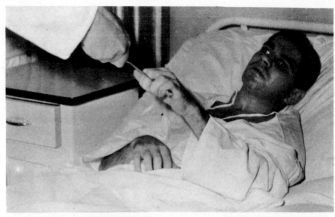
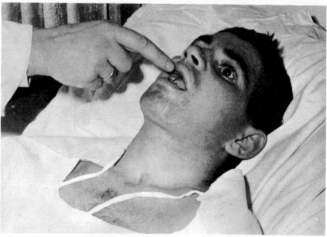

Fig. 16.—Grasp reflex ("magnetic reaction") and mouthing phenomenon in a patient with severe craniocerebral trauma. The patient grasps objects held before him—particularly objects held on the side opposite to the damaged frontal lobe—and refuses to release his fingers when asked to do so. When an object is shown to the patient and advances toward him, he opens his mouth. These signs signify the release of primitive, reflex mechanisms which often are reproducible.

Brain damage, irrespective of its cause, produces phenomena that indicate a release from higher control centers. The *snout phenomenon* (orbicularis oris reflex) is common: on light tapping with a finger or spatula at the corner of the mouth, the patient purses his lips. The *mouthing reflex* (sucking reflex) is less common and indicates more severe brain damage: the patient opens his mouth whenever an object is advanced toward it. The *grasp reflex* occurs with contralateral frontal lobe lesions and ipsilateral brainstem lesions: the patient grips objects firmly in his hand and fails to release them. This phenomenon is physiologic at birth and normally remains present during the first 2 months of life. A related sign is the compulsive grasping seen in patients with frontal-lobe lesions—they may seize and hold onto any passing object. The most important physical sign is the *Babinski sign:* this is a *sign of pyramidal tract damage,* consisting of tonic dorsiflexion of the great toe with simultaneous spreading of the other toes on firm stroking of the sole of the foot with a pointed object. The same toe and foot movement may be elicited by stimulating the skin in the groove behind the lateral malleolus *(Chaddock's sign),* by massaging the lower calf muscles *(Gordon's sign)* and after firm pressure along the surface of the shin *(Oppenheim's sign).* These phenomena may be spontaneous or crossed. In many infants up to the end of the first year of life, and sometimes up to the end of the second, they are physiologic. The Babinski sign is an easily elicitable and reliable sign of pyramidal tract damage. The first stage may be the appearance of nonreacting soles. *Decerebration* follows interruption of all impulses from the cerebrum to the periphery and vice versa at the level of the brain stem: the patient lies unconscious with arms extended (sometimes pronated), legs outstretched and eyes open. These extensor phenomena may increase on stimulation to become frank extensor spasms.

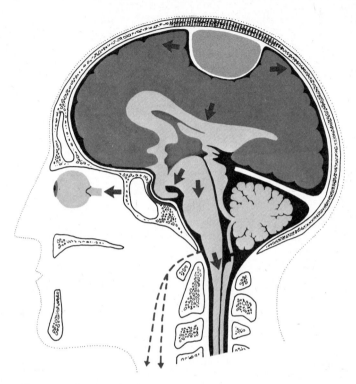

Fig. 17.—In this diagram, a meningioma of the parietal falx is utilized to illustrate the effects of an intracranial space-occupying mass lesion: focal bone erosion (or hyperostosis) is present and later the dorsum sellae of the pituitary fossa becomes atrophic. Later effects include: papilledema, displacement of the ventricular system, projectile vomiting and bradycardia due to vagal stimulation and mental changes due to increased intracranial pressure. The end result is coma and a decerebrate state due to caudal displacement of the brainstem and secondary brainstem hemorrhages.

Raised intracranial pressure can be produced by tumors, brain abscess, intracranial hematomas, infectious granulomas and cerebral edema. Focal symptoms (see p. 166) depend on the location of the mass; seizures occur early.

Space-occupying Intracranial Lesions (Syndrome of Raised Intracranial Pressure)

According to the Monro-Kellie doctrine, the sum of the volumes of brain, blood and cerebrospinal fluid remains constant.

Rapidly enlarging space-occupying intracranial lesions (tumors, hematomas, etc.) produce first a rise in pressure in the CSF compartment, then compression of the brain substance and finally failure of the cerebral blood supply. If operation is not performed, the raised intracranial pressure leads to headache, a *clouding of consciousness, coma* and *cerebral death (decerebration)*.

Lesions that grow more slowly produce a variety of effects: congestion of the optic nerves *(papilledema)*, pressure changes in the skull bones *("pressure sella"), prominent digital markings* and suture diastasis in children and adolescents, various cranial nerve palsies (abducens; *double vision* on lateral gaze; vagus: *projectile vomiting* without choking, especially during rapid head movements and brady- and tachycardia; 8th nerve: vertigo), eventually leading to the *syndrome of chronic raised intracranial pressure*. The patient becomes slowed, his insight is limited, affect and mood are altered and he is disoriented. EEG reveals a slowing of the background rhythm *(generalized changes);* carotid arteriography shows a prolonged circulation time. Without operation, tentorial herniation with extensor spasms ensues.

The final picture is that of an unconscious patient lying with arms flexed (seldom outstretched) and legs extended. The pupils, initially contracted, are widely dilated and fail to react to light; an attempt to elicit reflexes fails or merely aggravates the extensor spasms. *The midbrain syndrome*—the result of functional dissociation of the fore- and midbrain—may cause hyperthermia and hyperglycemia. Pressure effects on the medulla oblongata lead to respiratory and circulatory failure, finally cerebral death (decerebration).

No lumbar puncture if raised intracranial pressure suspected! Brain herniation may make it fatal!

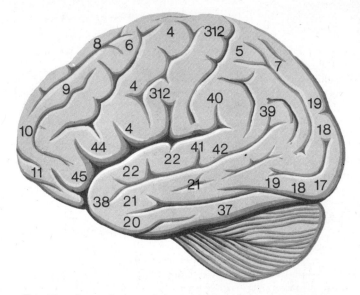

Fɪɢ. 18.—Lateral view of the cerebral cortex, indicating Brodmann's cytoarchitectonic fields. Area *4:* precentral region (motor cortex) with Betz cells. Areas *1, 2* and *3:* postcentral region (sensory cortex). Areas *17, 18* and *19:* visual cortex. Area *22:* auditory cortex. Area *44:* motor speech cortex (Broca's area). Ill-defined functional centers (see text): Areas *5* and *7:* astereognosis, amorphognosia, ahylognosia. Area *40:* apraxia. Area *39:* agraphia, alexia, acalculia, right-left disorientation, finger agnosia. Areas *41* and *42:* sensory (Wernicke's) aphasia. Area *20:* amusia. These centers, some of which are disputed and poorly defined, apply only to right-handed individuals! Amnestic aphasia (word blindness) usually is a symptom of a generalized cerebral disorder but occasionally it localizes the lesion to the temporoparietal region.

In about 90% of the human race, the so-called right-handers, the left cerebral hemisphere possesses a special significance for image formation, the understanding of symbols and language concepts— and therefore for speech. According to Broca, lesions of the lower and posterior part of the frontal lobe (Area 44) render the patient unable to utter despite intact motor machinery for speech *(motor aphasia)*. He says little and utters syllables and words that reveal a disturbance of word formation *(paraphasia)*.

Lesions of Area 22 cause difficulty in understanding speech (Wernicke). Patients with such lesions often are uncontrollably voluble or speak gibberish, and they fail to understand the spoken word, completely *(sensory aphasia)* or incompletely. In the presence of an extensive lesion of the left hemisphere, the ability to articulate and understand speech is completely lost. Motor and sensory speech disturbances are (nearly?) always combined—with differing degrees of emphasis in individual cases. Disturbances in word (concept) building and word (concept) understanding are also reflected in the patient's inability to read *(alexia)*, write *(agraphia)* and calculate *(acalculia)*. In such cases, a lesion of the more posterior part of the brain (Area 39 and vicinity) often is present. Correct body orientation may be lost *(autotopagnosia)* and the patient cannot tell left from right.

Lesions of the angular gyrus, typically characterized by *finger agnosia*, also produce an element of word blindness that careful examination will reveal. The above-named (and other) higher cerebral functions for synthesizing concepts and symbols are fully integrated. Topographic localization of these functions is difficult: although they correspond roughly to sensory and motor centers that occupy fixed locations in the cerebral cortex, precise anatomic localization is impossible.

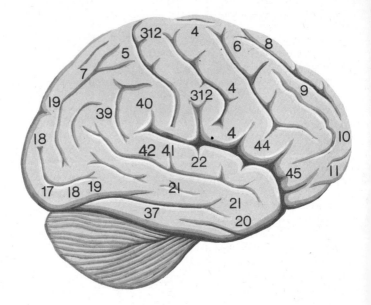

Fɪɢ. 19.—Lateral surface of right hemisphere: Area *4:* precentral region (motor cortex) with the following topographic localization: Pyramidal cells for the foot in the upper part, for the leg in the middle part, then for the arm and in the lowest part those for the head musculature. The use of this classification in Areas *1, 2* and *3* for a corresponding sensory "homunculus" is less clear-cut. The function of the right temporal lobe in right-handed individuals is uncertain. Areas *17, 18* and *19* represent the visual cortex. Areas *5, 7, 39* and *40* serve several complex functions, notably orientation (see text). Temporal lobe lesions of either hemisphere may cause homonymous hemianopia.

The higher cerebral functions of the right, i.e., nondominant, hemisphere in right-handed individuals (and, with certain limitations, the left hemisphere in left-handed ones) are not easily recognizable. However, the nondominant (right) hemisphere never is "silent": for example, lesions of the right parietal lobe impair spatial orientation. A feature is *disorientation of space,* which is clearly illustrated if the patient tries to draw simple maps or sketches—he loses his ability to sketch a bicycle or to build block designs *(constructional apraxia).* The patient has difficulty in carrying out fine hand movements that require a certain amount of concentration *(dressing apraxia).* Very often he neglects the opposite side, in the absense of a definite homonymous hemianopia. The latter may be suspected in a severely ill patient if sudden stimulation applied to one visual field evokes no response and the identical stimulus applied to the opposite field evokes a prompt response. In such cases, the contralateral field disturbance may be complex and difficult to analyze in individual cases. The lesion may be more clearly defined if the examiner obtains no response on addressing the patient from one side of his body, yet the patient immediately recognizes him and converses normally when he shifts to the opposite side. The patient may completely lose recognition of the side of the body opposite a lesion *(hemisomatognosia):* he views an arm or leg placed in a certain position as a foreign body. He may not be aware of his disease *(anosognosia).* Temporal lobe lesions of the nondominant hemisphere still are not satisfactorily classified, and they remain difficult to recognize. In left-handed individuals, spatial relationships are not well defined but the "speech center" usually (but not always) is in the right hemisphere. Parieto-occipital lesions produce faulty recognition of faces (prosopagnosia), objects and colors.

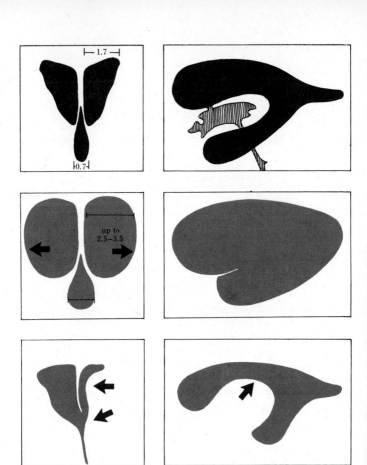

Fig. 20.—**(top)** Outline of a normal pneumoencephalogram. In the AP view, the lateral ventricles and 3rd ventricle are visible, and in the lateral view one sees the anterior, temporal and occipital horns, the 3rd ventricle, the aqueduct and the 4th ventricle. **(center)** Cerebral atrophy (hydrocephalus ex vacuo) and extraventricular obstructive hydrocephalus both enlarge the ventricular system: each lateral ventricle is wider than 1.7 cm and the 3rd ventricle larger than 0.7 cm. The impression of the basal ganglia is missing (→). **(bottom)** Space-occupying lesions displace and compress the ventricles. In the lateral view there may be an abnormal indention corresponding to a tumor outline (→).

Roentgenologic Examination of the Skull and Brain

Scout roentgenograms of the skull in AP and lateral projections may show evidence of chronically raised intracranial pressure: *"pressure sella," suture diastasis* (in children) and *increased digital impressions of the cranial vault. Focal space-occupying lesions* are indicated by contralateral pineal displacement, local hyperostosis or bone erosion (meningioma or metastases), calcified deposits (physiologic choroid plexus and falx "calcifications": oligodendroglioma or meningioma) and ballooning of the pituitary fossa in pituitary adenomas. *Fractures* are not always visible or distinguishable from vascular channels. A *geographic skull* suggests plasmacytoma. *Roentgenograms of the skull base* often are essential: they may reveal fractures or bone erosion, particularly widening of normal foramina (Schwannomas?). Suspicion of infratentorial or lesions at the base of the skull makes special views necessary: *Stenver's projection* will reveal widening of the internal auditory canal by cerebellopontine angle Schwannomas, and both this and Schuller's projection show destruction of the apex of the petrous pyramid in meningiomas, etc.

The course of the optic nerve is studied by special optic foramen views. *Frontal tomograms* are helpful for a side-to-side comparison on central structures at the skull base, e.g., the craniovertebral angle. Here, the dividing line between irrelevant normal variants and significant features often is difficult to define.

Pneumoencephalography

Fractional filling with 25–50 ml of air injected by the lumbar route (or 25–40 ml by cisternal injection) usually demonstrates the ventricular system adequately. Spot films can be made, with the aid of the image intensifier, of the aqueduct, 4th ventricle and basal cisterns. Disease processes may give rise to focal ventricular enlargement (atrophy), compression (local space-occupying process) or displacement (pressure effect of a treatable mass: tumor? abscess? hematoma?).

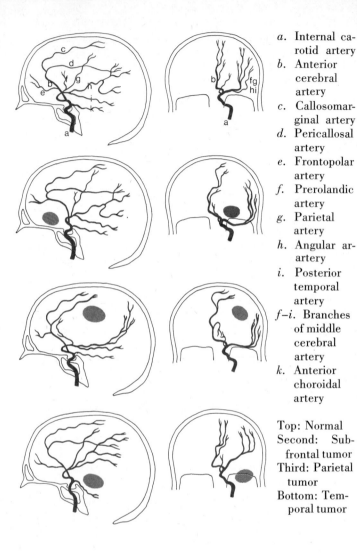

a. Internal carotid artery
b. Anterior cerebral artery
c. Callosomarginal artery
d. Pericallosal artery
e. Frontopolar artery
f. Prerolandic artery
g. Parietal artery
h. Angular arartery
i. Posterior temporal artery
f–i. Branches of middle cerebral artery
k. Anterior choroidal artery

Top: Normal
Second: Subfrontal tumor
Third: Parietal tumor
Bottom: Temporal tumor

Cerebral Angiography

Injection of the carotid artery in the neck demonstrates the carotid siphon and anterior and middle cerebral arteries, and in 10–20% of patients the posterior cerebral artery as well. Abnormalities to be observed include vascular occlusions, stenoses, displacements and abnormal vascularity (angiomas, *vascular meningiomas*, which stain uniformly, and glioblastomas, which evidence a "spider-web" circulation).

Significant pathologic findings are *arterial aneurysms*, which are most common on the anterior communicating artery (see p. 140).

Functional vascular narrowing, i.e., arterial spasm, may occur around the needle during carotid angiography and in the vicinity of aneurysms. Provided that the proper indications are observed (excluding the very old, severe hypertensives) and a satisfactory technique is followed (avoidance of subintimal injection or excessive volumes of contrast medium), the injection of 8–12 ml of contrast medium, e.g., sodium iothalamate, into the carotid artery (common or internal) is virtually harmless. Serial angiography is utilized to determine the speed of passage of the contrast bolus through the brain; slowing indicates raised intracranial pressure. In the *venous phase*, the thalamostriate vein outlines the lateral wall and floor of each lateral ventricle: dilatation of the ventricle displaces the vein downward and bows it. Early venous filling in tumors indicates arteriovenous shunting, usually a sign of malignancy. Avascular areas suggest hematomas, or avascular tumors (astrocytomas, oligodendrogliomas).

Vertebral angiography is especially important in demonstrating *aneurysms and arteriovenous malformations* of the posterior cranial fossa. Filling of the basilar artery and its branches and the posterior cerebral artery can be achieved by catheterization of the femoral artery (Seldinger). Interpretation requires considerable experience, in view of many normal variations. Compression of the basilar trunk against the clivus indicates the presence of a space-occupying process, especially in the cerebellar hemisphere or pons. Arteriovenous malformations and aneurysms usually are well visualized. Gliomas have less typical appearances.

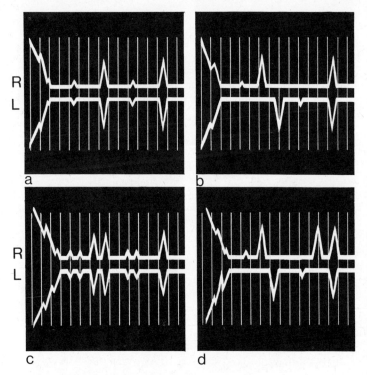

Fig. 22.—From right *(R)* and from left *(L)*, the initial echo, the lateral ventricle, the midline echo, the opposite lateral ventricle and the terminal echo are **(a)** normal. **(b)** Left-sided space-occupying lesion (midline echo displaced 0.9 cm to the right side). **(c)** Dilated ventricles, i.e., hydrocephalus (3rd ventricle wider than 0.8 cm.). **(d)** Left-sided space-occupying lesion with 0.7 cm displacement of midline echo and so-called hematoma echo (recognizable on recording from the right side).

Echoencephalography

Sound impulses transmitted at a frequency of 2 MHz from a piezoelectric crystal will be reflected by various fixed intracranial structures, such as the falx, septum pellucidum, ventricular walls, pineal, hematoma and some tumors. The transducer serves also as a receiver to record the reflex echoes, which are displayed on a cathode ray oscilloscope and may be recorded with a Polaroid camera. By measuring the bitemporal diameter of the patient before examination, the anticipated position of the midline echo can be calculated. It always is possible to identify the midline structures (displacement over 2 mm is pathologic), often the 3rd ventricle (normal 4–7 mm, often wider in elderly subjects). Sometimes the lateral ventricle, a tumor or a subdural hematoma may be visible. The most important *indication* for echoencephalography is to verify the position of the midline structures in unilateral space-occupying lesions by means of repeated measurements at short intervals— especially suspected *epidural or subdural hematomas*. In the course of excluding an intracranial tumor, echoencephalography enables space-occupying lesions of one hemisphere to be identified, and the method also furnishes evidence of obstructive hydrocephalus in infratentorial masses (diameter of 3rd ventricle greater than 0.8–1 cm).

Cerebral Scintigraphy

Certain radioisotopes (notably ^{197}Hg, ^{131}I, ^{99m}Tc) accumulate in the brain following intravenous injection and can be visualized by a scintillation counter. Tumors, any local breakdown in the bloodbrain barrier and vascular lesions are demonstrated as areas of increased activity. The precise localization of these lesions may be determined by lateral and A-P views. The technique does not harm the patient; he merely has to lie still on a couch. False positive as well as false negative results are encountered.

CT Scanning

Computer-assisted scanning of the brain (CAT, CT or EMI scanning) is a revolutionary imaging technique that provides a computer print-out, rather than a conventional roentgenogram, of axial skull tomography. The various intracranial structures possess different tissue densities that, when viewed in the print-out, provide a detailed and accurate picture of the brain. This new clinical method promises to supersede conventional neuroradiologic contrast methods in the diagnosis of space-occupying and some other intracranial lesions.

45

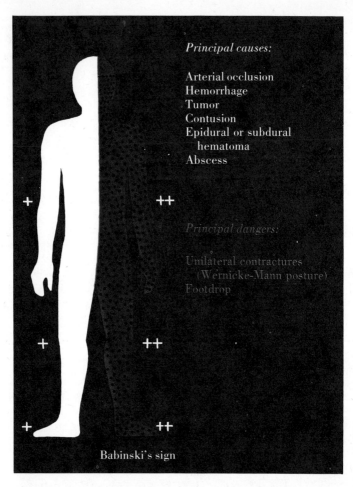

Principal causes:

Arterial occlusion
Hemorrhage
Tumor
Contusion
Epidural or subdural
   hematoma
Abscess

Principal dangers:

Unilateral contractures
   (Wernicke-Mann posture)
Footdrop

Babinski's sign

Fig. 23.—The most common topographic syndrome is contralateral hemiparesis or hemiplegia caused by damage to a cerebral hemisphere. Muscles of the forehead, throat and back are spared. Sensation may be diminished but the deficit does not reach the midline. Deep tendon reflexes are increased after the acute stage has passed; Babinski's sign is present. A lesion of the internal capsule (occlusion of the lenticulostriate artery) is a frequent cause.

46

The first part of the neurologic physical examination provides the topographic diagnosis. The predominating symptomatology will reveal the location of the disease. One speaks of:

Myopathies to describe purely muscle diseases.

Anterior horn (root) lesions—isolated diseases of the lower motor neuron.

Posterior root (radicular) lesions—segmental sensory disturbances.

Peripheral nerve palsies—combined motor and sensory deficits of neural type, with loss of reflexes.

Unilateral spinal cord lesions—dissociated unilateral disturbances of sensation with contralateral weakness.

Transection syndrome—complete sensory and motor loss below the lesion with disturbances of bladder and bowel function.

Spinocerebellar syndromes—unilateral or bilateral ataxia, asynergy, adiadochokinesia.

Extrapyramidal lesions—hyperkinesia, muscle rigidity, poverty of movement.

Raised intracranial pressure—papilledema, headache, vomiting, confusion and roentgenologic evidence of "pressure sella" and increased calvarial markings.

Epilepsy—occurrence of more than one generalized seizure, and the EEG shows paroxysmal activity.

Syndrome of the nondominant hemisphere—agnosia, constructional apraxia and anosognosia.

Posterior fossa syndrome—signs of raised intracranial pressure and cranial nerve palsies.

Brain stem syndrome—unilateral damage to cranial nerve nuclei and contralateral pyramidal tract involvement.

Meningeal syndrome—neck stiffness, pleocytosis, raised protein content in the CSF and pyrexia.

Midbrain syndrome—somnolence, tetraplegia and oculomotor palsy.

This classification is the basis of nosologic orientation in neurology.

Neurologic Status

Individual clinical findings, when grouped together, make up the neurologic status of the patient. This always should include the following details: Right- or left-handed—mobility of the head—nuchal rigidity? Blood pressure—both carotid pulses—bruits?

Cranial Nerves:

- I: Beeswax and vanilla detectable in both nostrils?
- II: Visual acuity—fundus—visual fields (properly corrected).
- III. Pupils: degree of dilatation—shape—light reaction—convergency reaction. Ocular movements directly upward and downward, inward and obliquely upward.
- IV: Ocular movements obliquely downward.
- V: Sensation—masticatory muscles—corneal reflex—masseter reflex—lacrimal secretion—taste sensation in anterior two-thirds of tongue.
- VI: Ocular movements outward.
- VII: Furrowing the forehead—facial muscles—whistling—hyperacusis—width of palpebral fissure—salivary secretion.
- VIII: Whispered speech—nystagmus.
- IX: Faucial sensation—taste sensation in posterior one-third of tongue—speech articulation.
- X: Uvula elevation—phonation—gag reflex.
- XI: Head turning—shoulder shrug.
- XII: Tongue protrudes normally? Atrophy? Fibrillation?

Arms:

Bulk 10 cm proximal and distal to the olecranon—power—sensation—tone—deep tendon reflexes: biceps (C5–6) triceps (C7–8), brachioradialis (C5–6)—sign of Hoffman.

Trunk:

Diaphragmatic breathing—sensation—rectus abdominis reflex—superficial abdominal reflexes—cremasteric reflex—sphincter ani reflex.

Legs:

Bulk 10 cm proximal and distal to the patella—power—sensation—tone—signs of Lasegue, Babinski, Rossolimo—deep tendon reflexes: adductors (L1–3), quadriceps (knee jerk, L2–4), triceps surae (ankle jerk, S1–2), tibialis posterior (L5)—defense mechanisms.

Coordination:
Gait—gait with eyes shut—deviation?—position of arms and co-ordination tests: finger—nose—knee—ankle—rapid alternating movements—Barany test—rebound phenomenon—writing sample.

Autonomic:
Vasomotor (dermatographism)—sudomotor (hyperhidrosis).

Mental Function:
Cooperation—orientation—dementia or disturbances of higher cortical function?

Neurologic Nosology

Topographic neurology is based on the principles of neuroanatomy and neurophysiology, and a knowledge of these disciplines is assumed. If this knowledge is present, topographic syndromes can be explained in general terms without reference to the nature of the disease.

Nosologic neurology is the vehicle for the first step, viz., integrating or classifying the disease into the framework of clinical medicine. It entails a review of the basic disease process and its etiology, and definition of its numerous relationships to other clinical specialties—to internal medicine, to ophthalmology, to otorhinolaryngology, to dermatology and to psychiatry. In all spheres, the link with surgery is close: a neurosurgeon is a neurologist utilizing special therapeutic methods.

In exploring the etiology of a topographically determined disease, further criteria need to be examined:

Hereditary disease may be revealed by careful history taking (questioning the relatives).

Infectious diseases may come to light through nonspecific signs of inflammation (high ESR, leukocytosis, pyrexia, etc.) and require bacteriologic, virologic and parasitologic investigation. It is important to obtain information about related illnesses in the community and infections due to animal bites—all contact with animals, details of foreign travels and earlier episodes of the same illness. Nearly all infectious agents and also the autoimmune diseases may affect the nervous system.

Diseases of blood vessels rarely are confined to the arteries and veins of the nervous system. Relevant facts are a history of previous myocardial infarction, transient difficulty in walking and underlying risk factors, such as hypertension, diabetes and hypercholesterolemia.

Neoplasms are confined to the CNS in about 75% of cases. However, every fourth brain tumor is a *metastasis* from a primary malignancy of the bronchus (51%), breast (9%), uterus (3%), rectum

(2.3%), prostate (1.7%), kidney (hypernephroma 5.3%), sarcoma or melanoma (frequencies according to Scheid). Chest roentgenograms and liver scans are useful in unexplained brain lesions to verify that the most important filters of metastases in the body are clear.

Metabolic disturbances (see p. 184) involve all systems. Direct proof of ganglion cell involvement is possible by biopsy of the rectal mucosa and of glial cell involvement by biopsy of the sural nerve. Failure of production of phytanic acid—the cause of *Refsum's disease* (polyneuritis, retinitis pigmentosa, ataxia and deafness)—may be discovered by examination of the blood. *Wilson's disease* is revealed by determining the serum copper and ceruloplasmin values, *hemosiderosis* of the brain by the serum iron level and *phenylketonuria* (inherited mental deficiency) by confirming the presence of excess phenylpyruvic acid in the urine by means of the ferric chloride test. Other inborn errors of metabolism may be revealed by paper chromatographic examination of 24-hour urine specimens. Deficiency of vitamin B_{12} and nicotinic acid *(pellagra)* exerts effects on the nervous system; also: diabetes mellitus (polyneuritis) and hypoglycemia (pancreatic islet-cell tumors may cause generalized seizures), uremia (polyneuritis, seizures, encephalopathy), liver diseases (encephalopathies), post-portacaval shunting syndrome (flapping tremor, *shunt encephalopathies* with dementia), porphyria (polyneuritis with encephalopathy), disturbances of endocrine and electrolyte metabolism and exogenous intoxications.

Trauma often is combined with fractures or injuries of the internal organs, which are detected by roentgenograms.

Malformations, either inherited or arising pre, peri- or postnatally, may affect other organs, e.g., heart, kidneys, skin and nails in tuberous sclerosis *(Bourneville-Pringle's disease)*. The diagnosis of other phakomatoses may be obvious on examination of the skin: café-au-lait patches and neuromata in *generalized neurofibromatosis* (von Recklinghausen), facial hemangiomata in the distribution of one trigeminal division of *Sturge-Weber's disease* and both retinal and *cerebellar hemangiomata in von Hippel-Lindau's disease*. In the *Louis-Bar syndrome*, cerebellar atrophy (ataxia, dysarthria!) is associated with telangiectases of the conjunctiva and external ear (pinna) and bronchiectasis.

All degenerative diseases of the CNS, indeed most disease processes affecting the brain, may be accompanied by *mental changes*. These may be mild and reversible or severe (organic brain syn-

52

dromes to coma). Also, the patient may show personality changes and irreversible diminution in intellectual capacity (dementia).

Thus, nosologic diagnosis requires the use of multidisciplinary investigative procedures and a constant contact with colleagues in other clinical specialties.

Treatment should be aimed *specifically* at eliminating or neutralizing the cause of the disease. Microorganisms can be dealth with by antibiotics, individual viruses by antiviral agents (herpes simplex with Ara A—adenosine arabinoside). Metabolic disturbances may respond to a correct diet and therapeutic drugs (in *Wilson's disease*, D-penicillamine). Blood vessel vasculitides should be treated by combating the edema, encouraging the development of the new collateral circulation and providing cardiac support (digitalis, strophanthin). Local tumors are treated by operative resection.

A vital part is played by *nonspecific therapy*. Complications may be prevented and lost function may be restored by supervised physiotherapy and electrotherapy of paralyzed muscles. In the peripheral nerves, complete regeneration is possible provided that some ganglion cells remain intact. In the CNS, the highly plastic state of the brain facilitates the transfer of functions to other parts that remain intact, by means of hitherto unutilized pathways.

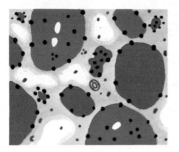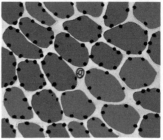

a

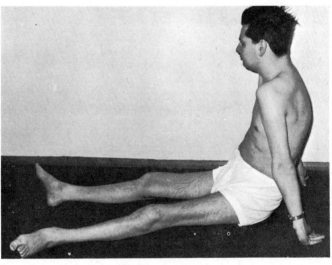

b

FIG. 24.—(a) *Left*, histologic section of muscle from a patient
with progressive muscular dystrophy, compared with normal muscle *(right)*. Individual fibers of normal size are separated by grossly
hypertrophied and atrophic fibers. Increased internal nuclei,
individual-fiber necrosis and fatty infiltration. (b) Patient with benign X-linked recessive muscular dystrophy. Severe weakness of
the pelvic and calf muscles, less severe involvement of other muscles. When the patient tries to stand up, the trunk is inched upward by the hands walking up the thighs (Gower's sign).

54

Myopathies

Etiology: Hereditary diseases, possible caused by hitherto un-recognized enzyme defects of muscle metabolism, or membrane defects.

Clinical: Increasing weakness and progressive degeneration of muscles over the course of years. The patient may remain mobile for a long time; he learns to use lever movements; "he clambers up himself from the seated to the erect position." The diseased muscles may hypertrophy through fatty infiltration ("pseudohyper-trophy"), especially the calves ("champagne bottle" legs) and involvement of the orbicularis oris muscles may lead to a pouting appearance of the lips ("tapir's mouth). The blood serum levels of the following enzymes are markedly raised: creatine phosphokinase, aldolase, LDH and other transaminases. The EMG shows typical low amplitude, brief, polyphasic motor-unit potentials. Electric excitability and the deep tendon reflexes remain normal for a long time.

Differential Diagnosis: In the absence of a clear-cut picture of hereditary disease, muscle biopsy is advisable: the typical picture comprises a mixture of hypertrophic fibers, degenerating fibers infiltrated by phagocytes, sarcolemmal rests rich in nuclei but devoid of myofibrils, fatty infiltration and some residual normal fibers.

The *Duchenne type* starts in the first years of life in the pelvic muscles, producing a hyperlordosis ("wasp-tail" deformity) and waddling gait ("duck's waddle"). *Trendelenburg's sign* is present: the erect patient stands on one leg and the pelvis tilts to the opposite side. Involvement of the leg, trunk, shoulder and arm muscles incapacitates the patient; often he dies of pneumonia before puberty. The disease is known to occur only in boys, being inherited as an X-linked recessive. Spontaneous mutations should be taken into account, the incidence being about 7 per 100,000 persons. Two other forms occur, the *Becker-Kiener type*, which is slowly progressive, and the *Emery-Dreifuss type*, which leads to early contractures. Both are sex-linked recessive diseases affecting the pelvic girdle muscles in boys and young men. A cardiomyopathy may be an additional finding.

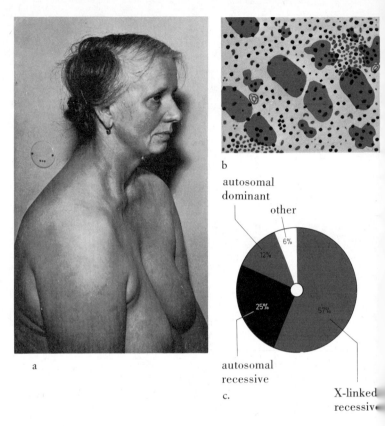

b

autosomal
dominant

other

6%

12%

25%

57%

autosomal
recessive

c.

X-linked
recessive

a

Fig. 25.—(a) Patient with facioscapulohumeral dystrophy. Both her son and brother also suffered from shoulder girdle weakness. The patient first noticed that she was unable to carry a bucket of water by her side—she had to carry it in front of her. (b) Histologic section of muscle in polymyositis. Lymphocyte and plasma cell infiltration in and between muscle fibers; later proliferation of connective tissue. (c) Incidence of various muscle dystrophies (according to Heyck and Laudahn).

56

Facioscapulohumeral dystrophy (*Erb-Landouzy-Dejerine* type) progresses very slowly. Inherited as an autosomal dominant, the disease commences in the shoulder girdle muscles: the trapezius, serratus anterior, rhomboid and pectoral muscles became involved first and the shoulder droops forward (winged scapula). The biceps muscle is severely affected, the triceps and deltoid muscles only mildly. Involvement of the facial muscles of expression produces the so-called myopathic facies. Later, the pelvic and leg muscles, especially the tibialis anterior, are affected. The disease may be overlooked for many years; often the changes are first observed by the patient's tailor. It is rare (4:1,000,000).

The *limb girdle type,* an autosomal recessive, is less rare (1:10,000?). Usually it commences in childhood and progresses more slowly. A rule in all the muscular dystrophies is that the proximal muscles are affected most severely. Exceptions *("distal"* and *"ocular" muscle dystrophies)* are known, occurring as autosomally inherited diseases in certain siblings.

Treatment: As long as the underlying metabolic defect remains unknown, no specific drug treatment can be offered. Physiotherapy may be beneficial: those muscle fibers remaining intact can be made to hypertrophy by isometric contraction exercises, and the risk of complications thus is reduced. Orthopedic intervention to prevent bone and joint deformities may be useful. A high-protein diet to prevent obesity is advisable.

In the "benign" forms of muscular dystrophy, the patient may continue to work for as long as 20 years.

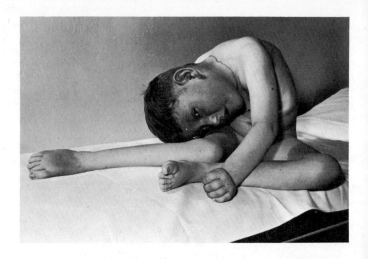

Fig. 26.—Severe muscle hypotonia from birth. Formerly called Oppenheim's disease, this condition is the result of various congenital myopathies, such as central core disease, nemaline myopathy, centronuclear myopathy and other diseases. The muscles are completely flaccid and possess no tone. The patient is unable to sit up unaided.

Muscle hypotonia, especially the floppy infant syndrome, has many other causes, such as early brain damage (pre-, peri- or postnatal damage) or an hereditary metabolic defect (see p. 191).

Polymyositis (Dermatomyositis)

Etiology: A collagen disease often overlooked, with or without skin lesions (see diagram, p. 56).

Clinical: Begins in the shoulder and back muscles, sometimes the pharyngeal or extremity muscles, which are reddened and painful. Step-like progression, with symptom-free intervals. Increasing muscle involvement eventually leads to considerable weakness. The diagnosis is suggested by generalized inflammatory changes (low grade fevers, accelerated ESR, leukocytosis and occasionally eosinophilia in the peripheral blood); confirmed by EMG, serum enzyme changes and muscle biopsy.

Treatment: Corticosteroids.

Congenital Myopathies

Become obvious soon after birth, particularly in the critical stage of motor development during infancy. Characterized by giant mitochondria, the accumulation of metabolic products in muscle fibers (central core myopathy) and rod-like structures at the margins of muscle fibers *(nemaline myopathy)* or by the persistence of embryonal elements *(myotubular myopathy)*. Muscle tone is markedly reduced and the child is very weak, but the disease does not appear to progress. Frequently familial.

Endocrine Myopathies

Proximal muscle weakness occasionally is seen in hyper- and hypothyroidism, Cushing's syndrome and hyperparathyroidism. The weakness diminishes after successful treatment of the underlying disease.

Toxic Myopathies

Proximal weakness may occur after *chloroquine, emetine,* prolonged *steroid* therapy and severe alcohol intoxications. *Chloroquine myopathy* leads to vacuolation and degeneration of type I muscle fibers.

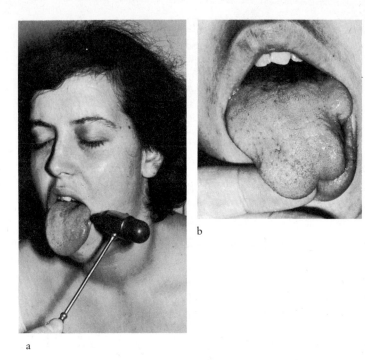

a

b

Fig. 27.—(a) Myotonic facies. Coarse rippling on tapping the tongue. (b) Snail-like contractions of the tongue in a myotonic patient after firm tapping. The trunk and extremity muscles bulged when tapped. The myotonic discharges produce a characteristic "dive-bomber" sound during electromyography.

MYOTONIA CONGENITA (THOMSEN'S DISEASE)

Etiology: Autosomal dominant disease, caused by decreased chloride conductance of the sarcolemma.

Clinical: The increased reactivity of the muscles leads to contractions, even on slight impulses or external stimulation (tapping). Although the muscles are large—the patient is often described as "muscle bound"—they contract slowly after having been at rest. Tapping provokes muscle bulging that continues for 10 seconds or more; the tongue shows pitting. Very weak currents can cause a contraction, a feature reflected in the EMG after voluntary activity as a burst of high-frequency potentials lasting several seconds— "dive-bomber" sound. Onset is often not recognized; the severity of the symptoms usually diminishes over the years.

MYOTONIC DYSTROPHY (CURSCHMANN-STEINERT'S DISEASE)

Etiology: Dominantly inherited common disease (5:10–100,000).

Clinical: Onset usually in middle age, sometimes in childhood, leading later to generalized muscle dystrophy affecting early type I fibers. The patient's face assumes an "expression of misery". Tapping of the muscles produces inconstant bulging lasting several seconds. The picture is completed by the mask-like facies (due to atrophy of the facial muscles), soft speech and myotonic reaction on electrical stimulation. In addition, testicular (ovarian) atrophy, frontal baldness and cataract are present. Despite slow progression of the disease, premature invalidism often is inevitable.

Treatment: Physiotherapeutic exercises to treat the diseased muscles. High-calorie, protein-rich diet.

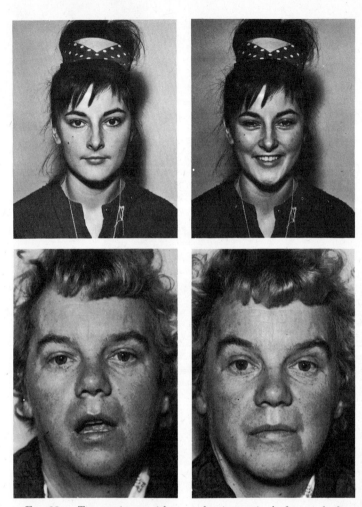

Fig. 28.—Two patients with myasthenia gravis, before and after injection of 10 mg of Tensilon. The face is mask-like, the mouth often hangs open. Approximately 90 seconds after injection, facial expression becomes normal and lasts for 2–3 minutes. The cause of this myopathic facies is a disturbance of impulse transmission at the motor end-plate.

Myasthenia Gravis

Etiology: A disturbance of the neuromuscular end-plate leading to progressively weaker muscle contractions, especially following prolonged activity. A prompt return to power follows the injection of Prostigmine (or Edrophonium, which acts in 1–3 minutes). These two substances block cholinesterase, thereby increasing acetylcholine at the neuromuscular junction. The disorder is caused by an autoimmune process directed against postsynaptic acetylcholine receptors. Two associations have been postulated, viz., either to the autoimmune diseases or to diseases of the thymus (thymic hyperplasia). A third association, viz., myasthenia gravis in intrathoracic tumors (carcinoma), is called the *Lambert-Eaton syndrome.*

Clinical: The characteristic feature is muscle weakness, which becomes obvious in the course of the day or after exertion; usually it is first observed in the muscles of the eyes, throat and jaw (choking, double vision), but other muscles may be affected also. The disease progresses in attacks, but inexplicable remissions occur. The patients usually are women around the age of 20 or 60 years. Electrical stimulation reveals a myasthenic reaction in the affected muscles; EMG shows a reduced amplitude after repetitive stimulation, which can be abolished by Tensilon. Inadequate treatment is dangerous—*myasthenic crisis,* when the patient may suffocate. Biopsy reveals no consistent recognizable lesion; occasionally a lymphocytic infiltration is present.

Treatment: Dosage with Prostigmine or a longer-acting drug such as Mestinon can be titrated to compensate completely for the disturbance of muscle power. Mestinon (60 mg) may be required up to 10 times a day, the individual doses being spaced according to individual requirements. Overdosage may produce a *cholinergic crisis* by depolarization of the motor end-plates—muscle weakness, spasm and twitching, dyspnea and hyperperistalsis. The diagnosis is confirmed if the patient's condition is aggravated by adding small doses of Tensilon; intravenous atropine then is indicated. Thymectomy has a favorable outcome in young patients or in those in whom the disease has been present for less than 2 years. Immunosuppressive therapy is useful.

Contraindicated (aggravation): Curare derivatives, quinine, phenothiazines, Valium, aminoglycoside antibiotics and magnesium.

Synopsis of Hereditary Myopathies (Modified from Walton: *Disorders of Voluntary Muscle*, 1974)

Name	Age at Onset	Variety	Inheritance
Duchenne's muscular dystrophy	3–5	pelvic girdle	X-linked recessive
Becker-Kiener muscular dystrophy	5–20	pelvic girdle	X-linked recessive
Emery-Dreifuss muscular dystrophy	4–5	pelvic girdle, with early contractures	autosomal recessive
Limb-girdle muscular dystrophy		pelvic and shoulder girdles	autosomal recessive
Facioscapulohumeral muscular dystrophy	10–30	shoulder, face	autosomal dominant
Congenital muscular dystrophy	at birth		
Distal muscular dystrophy	40–60	hands, ankles	autosomal dominant
Ocular muscular dystrophy (pharyngeal)	23–40	extraocular muscles, pharynx	dominant
Central core disease (Shy-Magee)	1	shoulder girdle, etc.	autosomal dominant
Rod body myopathy (Shy, Engel, *et al.*)	1	shoulder girdle, hypotonia	autosomal dominant
Myotubular myopathy (Spiro *et al.*)	early	shoulder girdle, hypotonia	
Megaconial and pleoconial myopathy	early	proximal paralysis	
Myotonia dystrophica	(3–)30	diffuse, baldness, cataract, testicular (ovarian) atrophy	autosomal dominant
Glycogenoses types II–VII	usually late childhood	diffuse, hypotonic (cardiac and hepatic involvement)	autosomal recessive

Rare myopathies include the muscle weakness accompanying disturbances of potassium metabolism (both *hyper-* and *hypokalemia*, occasionally also seen in normokalemic states), which are paroxysmal in nature, appearing suddenly and lasting for hours. They occur at rest after strenuous exercise, after exposure to cold and after high-carbohydrate meals. The hypokalemic form responds promptly to potassium intake.

Inherited phosphorylase deficiency *(McArdle's disease)* is caused by defective catabolism of glycogen. It is characterized by painful muscle spasms and weakness. Physical exercise produces no rise in the lactic acid level of the venous blood. *Rhabdomyolysis* with sudden *myoglobinuria* may follow strenuous exertion, various intoxications, anesthesia in *malignant hyperpyrexia* and occasionally McArdle's disease. *Neuromyotonia* is a term applied to increasing spasms of the skeletal musculature, which can be abolished by diphenylhydantoin.

Treatment: Diazepam.

Differential Diagnosis of Myopathic and Neurogenic Diseases

	Myopathy	*Neuropathy*
Clinical:	Proximal atrophy more common	Distal atrophy
	Sensory disturbances absent	Sensory deficits almost always present
	Deep tendon reflexes retained until late	Reflexes disappear early
	Skin seldom abnormal	Vaso-sudo-pilo-motor disturbances
	Only local pain	Nerve pressure and pain on stretching
	Normal chronaxy	Increased chronaxy
EMG:	Complete interference pattern with low amplitude of individual potentials. These are smaller, may be polyphasic	Larger and longer duration individual potentials; fibrillation potentials and positive sharp waves, incomplete interference pattern on maximal innervation
Histology:	All stages of degenerative changes combined: central nuclei, basophilia, nuclear enlargement, vacuolated fibers, necrosis of individual fibers, proliferation of connective and fatty tissues. "String of pearls" nuclear arrangement. Hypertrophy of individual fibers	Atrophy of specific groups of muscle fibers, with only slight degenerative changes. Often preferential involvement of type II muscle fibers ("white fibers"). Contrasted with groups of normal fibers are groups showing an identical degree of advanced atrophy

| Enzymology: | Creatine phosphokinase, SGOT, SGPT and LDH slightly or markedly elevated | Creatine phosphokinase, SGOT, SGPT and LDH normal or only slightly elevated |

Diseases of Cranial and Peripheral Nerves

Very few nerves are purely motor or purely sensory. The clinical picture common to nearly all peripheral nerve lesions is a combination of flaccid muscle weakness, atrophy and abnormal electrical conductivity with sensory and vaso-sudo-pilo-motor disturbances in the distribution of the affected nerve (see p. 13). The deficits are most clearly present in the *autonomous zone* of the nerve; along the peripheral margins, due to overlapping innervation, they may be recognized less easily.

Etiology: A wide spectrum of diseases cause peripheral nerve damage—all the disease entities so far discussed in this book may be responsible. The two most common are traumatic damage and toxic agents.

Diagnosis: This is reached by assessing subjective complaints and the extent of the motor, sensory and autonomic deficits and determining the presence or absence of chronaxy and the nerve conduction time. Muscle or nerve biopsy (e.g., sural nerve) only rarely will be necessary—the latter on the suspicion of a glial disease *(leukodystrophy)*. Circumferential measurements of muscle mass for side-to-side comparison and serial follow-up examination should be done.

Treatment: This is directed at the cause of the nerve disease. *Neurotmesis* requires nerve suturing; *axonotmesis* may respond to relocation operations on the damaged nerve: pressure from a hematoma, fracture fragment, a fibrous band or a stenotic segment along its course ("entrapment")—facial canal, olecranon, supinator canal or carpal or tarsal tunnel—may delay or prevent regeneration.

Nonspecific measures (seé p. 99), carried out on the damaged second neuron, are essential. The musculature may be preserved by means of physiotherapy and *electrical stimulation* during the long period required for nerve regeneration. Depending on the length of the damaged nerve and the extent of the damage, this period may vary between 6 months and 2 years (see p. 98).

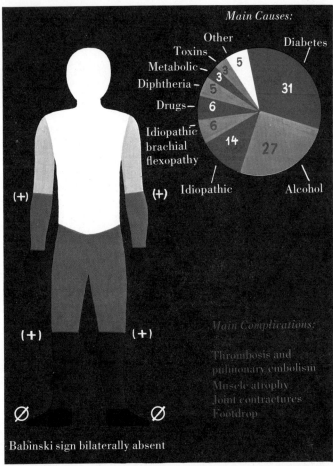

Babinski sign bilaterally absent

FIG. 29.—Clinical picture, etiology and main complications of the polyneuropathies. Usual findings include distal weakness and sensory disturbances, hypotonic muscles and absent reflexes. Later, neurogenic muscle atrophy follows. Asymmetric polyneuropathies ("mononeuritis multiplex") are seen with periarteritis nodosa, neuralgic amyotrophy, lead poisoning (radial palsy), serum injections (shoulder, also peroneal palsy) and occasionally with diabetes. Percentage frequency of neuropathies according to Neundörfer.

Pathology: Patchy degeneration of myelin sheaths and axis cylinders, lymphocytic and plasma cell infiltration are present, followed later by a proliferation of Schwann cells and endo- and perineurium, and shrinkage, vaculolation and degeneration of ganglion cells.

Etiology: Intoxications (arsenic, lead, thallium, ethanol, triorthocresylphosphate, carbon disulfide), *therapeutic drugs* (INH – prevented by vitamin B_6 administration; nitrofurantoin; thalidomide; perhaps also methaqualone — in chronic overdosage; vincristine; some antibiotics), *diabetes, porphyria, uremia,* malabsorption, hepatic cirrhosis, dysproteinemias, *periarteritis nodosa,* serum sickness and infections (diphtheria, leprosy, typhus, botulism, etc.). Many cases remain unexplained *("idiopathic polyneuropathy").*

Clinical: Symptoms begin distally and spread proximally, i.e., "rising." They comprise typically: paresthesias, hypesthesias, muscle weakness and absent reflexes; later, pseudoataxia, paralysis, vasomotor paralysis and muscle atrophy. They appear in the course of days or weeks. Chronaxy is prolonged, rheobase is increased, nerve conduction is reduced. The CSF protein is slightly raised — except in *idiopathic polyneuritis (Guillain-Barré syndrome),* in which it may be very high *(albumino-cytologic dissociation).* Removal of the causal factor always leads, within a few months, to regression of the clinical features — in the reverse order of their appearance. The main risks are *respiratory paralysis* and *thrombosis* due to stasis in the pelvic and extremity veins caused by physical inactivity — often lead to fatal *pulmonary embolism;* also footdrop and intramuscular fibrous tissue proliferation.

Diagnosis: Chronic progressive forms may be confused with spinal muscular atrophies, hereditary peroneal muscular atrophy and *Dejerine-Sottas polyneuropathy.* Acute forms may be mistaken for periodic paralysis.

Treatment: Removal of the causal factor and the prevention of complications is essential: controlled (assisted) ventilation, correct positioning in bed, physiotherapy, electrical stimulation, prevention of thrombosis (anticoagulants?).

Polyneuritides with a lymphocytic meningitis may complicate echo-, arbo- virus and coxsackievirus infections.

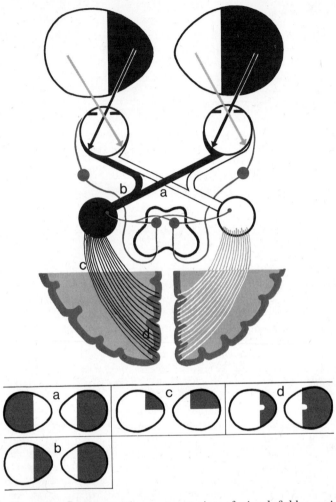

Fig. 30.—Diagrammatic representation of visual fields, optic pathways, and pathway subserving papillary reflex. Below, typical lesions: **(a)** Bitemporal hemianopia (chiasmal lesion). **(b)** Homonymous hemianopia (lesion in optic tract). **(c)** Quadrantic hemianopia (lesion in optic radiations). **(d)** Hemianopia with macular sparing.

70

LESIONS OF THE CRANIAL NERVES

Olfactory (1st cranial nerve, actually a part of the brain)

An olfactory nerve lesion may be assumed when the patient is able to identify substances used for trigeminal testing but not those for smell. Great variations are found among individuals in their ability to recognize olfactory test substances. *Anosmia* following craniocerebral trauma suggests rupture of the olfactory filaments and, if spontaneous, a *meningioma of the olfactory groove* (cribriform plate). Olfactory hallucinations indicate a lesion in the vicinity of the uncus ("uncinate fits").

Optic (2d cranial nerve, actually a tract of the brain)

Etiology: Blindness or deterioration of vision affecting the entire visual field, unilateral or bilateral, being caused by a retrobulbar neuritis (idiopathic, an early sign of multiple sclerosis, following *methyl alcohol abuse*, or vitamin B_{12} deficiency states), vascular obstruction (central retinal artery occlusion or venous thrombosis) or an *optic glioma* (also accompanying *tuberous sclerosis*). Intracranial space-occupying lesions tend to cause *papilledema*, i.e., congestion of the optic discs. *Optic atrophy*—easily recognizable by the blanched appearance of the disc—may complicate all the above-named lesions; also *tabes dorsalis* or it may represent *familial optic atrophy (Leber's disease)*. *Arachnoiditis of the opticochiasmatic cistern* is another cause. Unilateral optic atrophy and contralateral papilledema *(Foster Kennedy syndrome)* is a rare mode of presentation of an ipsilateral frontal tumor. *Meningioma of the tuberculum sellae* produces partial blindness, which may progress to optic atrophy. *Bitemporal defects of the visual fields* point to a pituitary lesion with suprasellar extension, damaging only the crossing fibers from the nasal half of both retinas. A *homonymous hemianopia* places the lesion in the optic tract, a *superior quadrantic homonymous hemianopia* localizes it to Meyer's loop (temporal region) and a homonymous hemianopia with sparing of macular vision to the calcarine region. Various local lesions may be responsible. Ischemia in the territory of the internal carotid artery may cause transient ipsilateral retinal blindness (emboli to ophthalmic artery: amaurosis fugax).

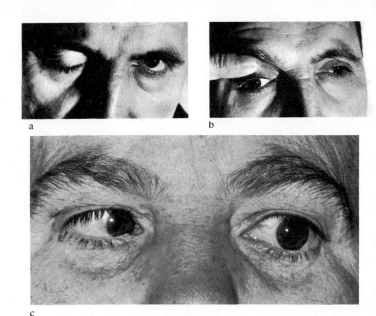

Fig. 31.—**(a)** Oculomotor palsy, indicated by right ptosis. **(b)** On lifting the eyelid, the right eyeball is seen to be deviated laterally (by the intact abducens nerve), causing diplopia. The pupil is dilated and unreactive. **(c)** Left abducens palsy. Outward rotation of the eyeball is impossible. Horizontal diplopia.

Oculomotor (3d cranial nerve)

Etiology: A lesion in the vicinity of the nucleus may be caused by infection (*syphilis, multiple sclerosis*, etc.), glioma, arteriovenous malformation, trauma, circulatory disturbances (*Weber's syndrome:* alternating hemiplegia with oculomotor palsy and contralateral hemiplegia due to pyramidal tract damage) or the pressure changes accompanying tentorial herniation (midbrain syndrome); the nerve may be damaged at the base of the brain by meningitis (TB), sarcoma, carcinoma (with unilateral involvement of all the lower cranial nerves—the so-called *Guillain-Garcin syndrome* or *hemibasal syndrome* [Kretschmer] or with paralysis of the 4th, 5th and 6th cranial nerves, *Jacod's syndrome*), also aneurysms. The *superior orbital fissure syndrome*, i.e., trochlear and abducens palsy with sensory loss in the distribution of the ophthalmic division of the trigeminal, accompanies lesions of the skull base or orbit (tumors, inflammatory lesions, etc.). Another cause is compression of the occulomotor nerve against the clivus by a space-occupying lesion.

Clinical: The globe is displaced forward and slightly downward; medial, lateral and upward movements become impossible. *Ptosis,* widely dilated pupil not reacting to light. If only the small gray nucleus *(Westphal-Edinger)* is affected, the pupil is dilated; if only the medial nucleus *(Perlia)*, the pupil fails to react to accommodation.

Trochlear (4th cranial nerve)

Isolated damage of the *infranuclear, crossed* fibers of the nerve is rare. (See also 3d cranial nerve.) Downward gaze (in adduction) is impaired.

Abducent (6th cranial nerve)

Etiology: Nuclear and nerve lesions as in oculomotor palsy. Circulatory disturbances *(Foville's syndrome)* additionally cause pyramidal tract syndromes (alternating hemiplegia: abducens palsy and contralateral hemiparesis). Early damage to the abducens nerve occurs in basal meningitides (TB) and in *Gradenigo's syndrome* with trigeminal involvement due to otogenic inflammation. *Fractures of the skull base* usually involve also the facial nerve.

Clinical: Lateral gaze is impaired, with a corresponding horizontal diplopia.

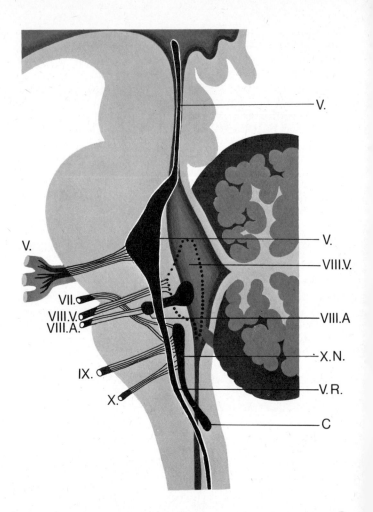

Fig. 32.—Diagrammatic cross section through the brain stem to show the nuclei of the sensory cranial nerves. The trigeminal nucleus usually is large and possesses long roots. The position of the vestibular nuclei is shown in dotted outline, since it lies more laterally. Acoustic neuromas, which usually arise from the vestibular nerve, deform the brain stem, 4th ventricle and cerebellum.

Trigeminal (5th cranial nerve)

Etiology: Diseases in the vicinity of the trigeminal nucleus— similar to oculomotor palsy, but rarer. Neuromas of the trigeminal nerve (cerebellopontine angle tumors) occur. The trigeminal nerve may be damaged in cerebellopontine angle tumors arising from schwannomas of the vestibular nerve. Meningitides, aneurysms and tumors of the base of the skull may damage it. A trigeminal deficit may accompany fracture of the facial bones.

Clinical: Sensory disturbances of the frontal, maxillary and mandibular nerves dominate the clinical picture. Muscle paralysis due to involvement of the masseter nerve is less frequent. The symptoms of paroxysmal pain in *trigeminal neuralgia* are important. The maxillary and mandibular divisions commonly are affected, usually in elderly subjects. Characteristically, the pain strikes like lightning, is very severe and disappears promptly ("tic douloureux"). The patient may be able to provoke an attack by touching certain areas ("trigger zones"). The etiology is not certain. Pain attacks may follow one and other.

Treatment: Trigeminal neuralgia often may respond to medium or large doses of anticonvulsants such as diphenylhydantoin or carbamazepine. Therapy-resistant cases: electrocoagulation of the Gasserian ganglion, retroganglionic neurotomy, etc.

Facial (7th cranial nerve)

Etiology: Various diseases in the vicinity of the facial nucleus may damage the nerve (see oculomotor palsy). Circulatory disorders cause the *Millard-Gubler syndrome:* facial palsy with contralateral hemiparesis due to a lesion involving the facial nucleus and ipsilateral pyramidal tract. *Bell's palsy* (idiopathic facial palsy) is the most common lesion of the facial nerve; others include otitic herpes zoster, and the *Melkersson-Rosenthal syndrome.* Facial nerve involvement is also a feature of *sarcoidosis, fracture of the base of the skull* and otogenic lesions. It may be involved in *vestibular (acoustic) schwannomas* (cerebellopontine angle tumor).

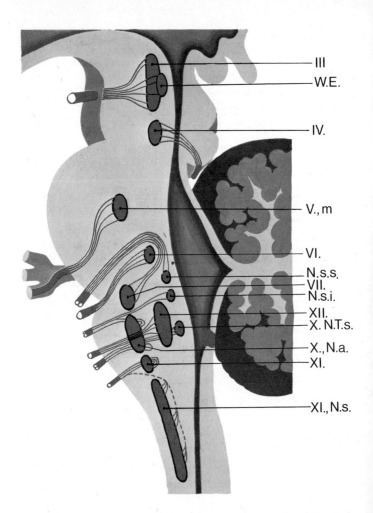

III

W.E.

IV.

V., m

VI.

N.s.s.
VII.
N.s.i.
XII.
X. N.T.s.
X., N.a.
XI.

XI., N.s.

Fig. 33. — Diagrammatic representation of the nuclei of the motor cranial nerves and the Westphal-Edinger nuclei, which mediate the pupillary light reaction. The vagus emerges from in the nucleus of the tractus solitarius *(X.N.T.s.)* and the nucleus ambiguus *(X.N.a.)*. In the floor of the 4th ventricle are the nucleus salvitorius

Clinical: Paralysis of the forehead and all the ipsilateral facial muscles, the stapedius (producing hyperacusis) and the platysma (test by protruding the chin and showing the teeth): the patient is unable to furrow his brow, shut the affected eye, puff out the cheeks or whistle. The chorda tympani, which traverses the tympanic cavity, may be damaged also, leading to absence or impairment of the sense of taste (ageusia, hypogeusia) in the ipsilateral anterior two-thirds of the tongue. Involvement of the greater superficial petrosal nerve, which carries parasympathetic fibers, causes an abnormal production of tears and saliva on the affected side. For prognosis, it is important to demonstrate chronaxy.

Treatment: Anti-inflammatory, anti-edema measures—i.e., corticosteroids in tapering doses. If recovery is not prompt, operative release of the nerve from the facial canal should be considered. Otherwise, treat according to etiology and the therapeutic demands of all peripheral nerve lesions. Nerve stimulation!

Auditory. Vestibular (8th cranial nerve)

Etiology: Various cerebral lesions may cause nuclear damage (see oculomotor palsy). Lesions at the base of the brain (meningitis, carcinoma, sarcoma) sometimes may be responsible. The most common is vestibular schwannoma (commonly and incorrectly called acoustic neuroma). Toxic damage due to streptomycin also occurs.

Clinical: The main symptoms are diminished hearing, sometimes amounting to deafness, and vertigo. In this area, neurology and otology overlap. *Ménière's syndrome* consists of attack of rotatory vertigo, which are heralded by vomiting and which last for hours; hearing is diminished. Between attacks, the patient is symptom-free. Nystagmus to the opposite side usually is observed. The cause is not known; hydrops of the semicircular canals may be responsible.

---

superior *(N.s.s.)* and inferior *(N.s.i.)*. The accessory nerve has a spinal root *(XI.N.s.)*. The trochlear nerve *(IV.)* crosses after emerging behind the colliculi.

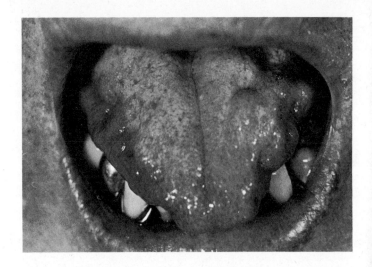

Fig. 34.—Atrophy of the left side of the tongue due to a lesion in the region of the hypoglossal nucleus. Atrophy of right lateral border is also visible. The two hypoglossal nuclei lie so close together that lesions involving the one usually affect the other. Paralysis of the orbicularis oris muscle accompanies hypoglossal nuclear damage and distinguishes these lesions from peripheral involvement of the hypoglossal nerve.

Glossopharyngeal (9th cranial nerve)

Etiology: Inflammatory, vascular, neoplastic and other disease processes may be responsible. The glossopharyngeal nerve as well as the 10th cranial nerve is involved by lesions of the jugular foramen, 10th and 11th *(Siebenmann's syndrome)* and virtually all the lower cranial nerves on one side in the so-called *hemibasal syndrome*. *Collet-Sicard's syndrome*, i.e., glosso-laryngo-scapulo-pharyngeal hemiplegia due to a complete lesion of the 9th, 10th, 11th and 12th cranial nerves, often is caused by a carcinoma or sarcoma of the base of the skull. In *Vernet's syndrome*, the ipsilateral glossopharyngeal nerve and pyramidal tract are involved (contralateral hemiplegia), due to a vascular accident.

Clinical: Clinical signs of nerve damage consist of unilateral sensory loss over the posterior pharyngeal wall and posterior one-third of the tongue and an incomplete palatal paralysis. The vomiting reflex is lost. *Glossopharyngeal neuralgia*, similar to trigeminal neuralgia, can be provoked by stimulation of trigger zones (gums, upper pharynx). Trigger zone: tonsillar region.

Vagus (10 cranial nerve)

Etiology: A variety of lesions of the medulla oblongata may be responsible. Vagal paralysis may be combined with glossopharyngeal palsy (see above). "Idiopathic." An indication of vagal involvement in bulbar palsy is paralysis of the recurrent laryngeal nerve, disordered phonation (the vowels i and e cannot be pronounced clearly) and hoarseness. Ipsilateral palatal palsy. Neuralgia of the auricular twig of the nerve causes sudden attacks of suboccipital pain; very rare!

Accessory (11th cranial nerve)

Etiology: Lesions of the medulla oblongata, jugular foramen (see above) and posterior cranial fossa, as well as peripheral lesions following biopsy of lymph nodes along the posterior margin of the sternomastoid muscle.

Clinical: Paralysis of the sternomastoid and upper part of the trapezius muscles, with a winged scapula and positional deformity of the shoulder. Weakness of head rotation.

Hypoglossal (12th cranial nerve)

Etiology: Lesions of the medulla oblongata and skull base. Idiopathic as in *bulbar palsy*. In *Jackson's syndrome*, associated with contralateral hemiparesis (alternating hemiplegia).

Clinical: Unilateral paralysis and hemiatrophy of the tongue. Paralysis of the orbicularis oris accompanies damage to the nucleus of the nerve.

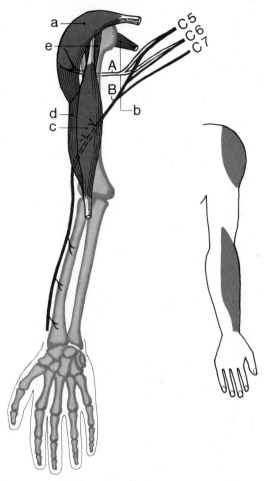

Fig. 35.—The axillary nerve *(A)*, arising from the C5 and C6 roots of the brachial plexus, supplies the deltoid *(a)* and teres minor *(b)* muscles. If the nerve is damaged, the patient is unable to raise his arm in a forward direction; external rotation of the shoulder is weak and there is a patch of sensory loss over the deltoid. In lesions of the musculocutaneous nerve *(B)*, arising from the C5–C7 roots,

80

Diseases of Peripheral Nerves (Paralyses)

Dorsal Scapular Nerve (from C4–5 roots)

Etiology: Isolated; very rarely involved in stab or gunshot wounds.

Clinical: The nerve supplies the levator scapulae and the rhomboids. The scapula assumes a characteristic deformity: its inferior angle is rotated outward and its medial border is raised from the posterior chest wall (winged scapula). The diagnosis is simple: the patient, in the prone position, is told to fold his arms behind his back. Without this maneuver, the lesion may pass unrecognized.

Suprascapular Nerve (from C4–6 roots)

Etiology: Isolated, in stab, slash or gunshot wounds. Rarely, the nerve is damaged during physical activities such as gymnastics or bricklaying, and it may complicate a fracture of the neck of the scapula.

Clinical: Paralysis of external rotation of the shoulder (supra- and infraspinatus muscles), weakness of arm raising in the course of external rotation. "A patient with suprascapular paralysis is unable to scratch the back of his head" (Mumenthaler).

Long Thoracic Nerve (C5–7)

Etiology: Weight-bearing pressure (back packs), a blow across the shoulders, violent shoulder movements. Isolated damage is also common in the course of resection of axillary lymph nodes or thoracotomy.

Clinical: Paralysis of serratus anterior muscle. The scapula is raised from the posterior thoracic wall, lies too close to the vertebral column and the inferior angle is rotated toward the midline. The deformity is accentuated by lifting the patient's arms forward.

---

the patient is unable to flex his elbow or supinate the forearm properly, due to weakness of the biceps *(c)*, brachialis *(d)* and coracobrachialis *(e)* muscles.

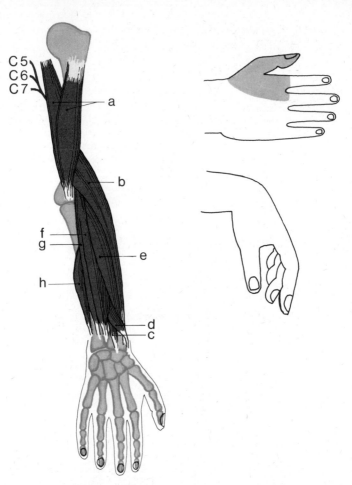

Fig. 36—**(Left)** Paralysis of the radial nerve affects the following muscles: *(a)* triceps brachii and anconeus, *(b)* brachioradialis, *(c)* extensors carpi radialis longus and brevis, *(d)* extensors pollicis longus and brevis, *(e)* abductor pollicis longus, *(f)* extensor indicis, *(g)* extensor digitorum communis and *(h)* extensor carpi ulnaris. The patient is unable to extend the wrist or the fingers. Supination of the forearm is restricted. **Top right,** cutaneous innervation of radial nerve. **Bottom right,** wrist drop of radial palsy.

Axillary Nerve (C5–6) (see Fig. 35, p. 80)

Etiology: Isolated damage accompanies anteroinferior dislocation of the shoulder joint or fracture of the surgical neck of the humerus; also sometimes after careless positioning, e.g., during general anesthesia.

Clinical: Deltoid palsy. Restriction of forward elevation of the arm, shoulder abduction and backward circumduction of the raised arm. Sensation is defective along the outer aspect of the shoulder and over the proximal part of the upper arm.

Musculocutaneous Nerve (C5–7) (see p. 80)

Etiology: Isolated damage is rare, following stab, slash or gunshot wounds. Local pressure is another cause; also iatrogenic injury in the course of operative repair of recurrent dislocation of the shoulder.

Clinical: Paralysis of the coracobrachialis, biceps and brachialis muscles; weakness of forward elevation of the arm and flexion when the arm is supinated. Sensation is defective on the radial side of the forearm as far as the base of the thenar eminence.

Radial Nerve (C5–7)

Etiology: The main causes of paralysis of the radial nerve or its branches are pressure effects (crutches, "Saturday night palsy," etc.), fractures of the humeral shaft, dislocation of the radial head and compression of the deep motor branch in the supinator canal.

Clinical: Upper radial damage, which is less common, causes weakness of the following muscles (Fig. 36): a. triceps brachii, b. brachioradialis, c. extensors carpi radialis longus and brevis, d. extensors pollicis longus and brevis, e. abductor pollicis longus, f. extensor indicis, g. extensor digitorum communis and h. extensor carpi ulnaris.

So-called *middle radial palsy* affects muscles b–h listed above: the patient has a wrist drop and is unable to abduct his thumb. In so-called *lower radial palsy,* muscles d–h are paralyzed. Damage to the deep (terminal) branch of the radial nerve—the *supinator canal syndrome*—paralyzes the extensor muscles of the third, ring and little fingers. Cutaneous sensation is defective or absent on the radial side of the back of the hand and thumb.

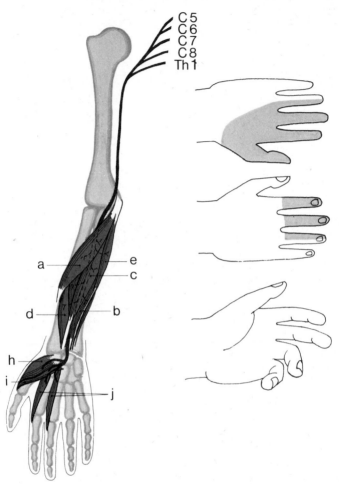

Fig. 37.—**(Left)** The median nerve arises from C5–T1 roots of the brachial plexus and supplies: *(a)* pronator teres, *(b)* the superficial and medial parts of the deep flexors of the fingers, *(c)* flexor carpi radialis, *(d)* flexor pollicis longus, *(e)* palmaris longus, pronator quadratus, opponens pollicis, *(h)* abductor pollicis brevis, *(i)* part of flexor pollicis brevis and *(j)* the 1st and 2d lumbrical muscles. Median paralysis prevents pronation of the forearm, palmar

Cheiralgia paresthetica is an isolated sensory deficit on the lateral side of the terminal digit of the thumb, heralded by pain and caused by damage to the terminal lateral branch of the superficial radial nerve (see p. 65).

Median Nerve (C5–T1)

Etiology: The main causes of damage to the median nerve are fracture of the humerus, external pressure (weight of the head of the sleeping partner—"lovers' paralysis"), fracture of the forearm bones, a stab wound at the wrist and compression beneath the transverse ligament of the wrist (carpal tunnel syndrome).

Clinical: In *upper median palsy,* the following muscles are affected: (1) pronator teres, (b) flexor digitorum superficialis and the radial half of flexor digitorum profundus, (c) flexor carpi longus and flexor radialis, (d) flexor pollicis longus, (e) palmaris longus, (f) pronator quadratus, (g) opponens pollicis, (h) abductor pollicis brevis, (i) the superficial head of flexor pollicis brevis and (j) the first and second lumbrical muscles. So-called *middle medial palsy* (muscles f–j) and distal median palsy (muscles g–j) affect mainly the thumb muscles. Through loss of abduction, the patient is unable to grasp a round object *("positive bottle sign")* and the thenar eminence is atrophic. The so-called *oath hand* is typical of proximal median palsy—the patient cannot flex his hand or index or middle fingers completely. The *carpal tunnel syndrome* is attributed to prolonged unilateral occupational strain producing local pressure at the wrist: starting as a nocturnal brachial paresthesia, it may progress to paralysis and atrophy of the thenar muscles; there is no sensory loss. The diagnosis is confirmed by nerve conduction measurements. Sensory disturbances in median palsy involve the medial half or the palm of the hand and the palmar surface of the index, middle and the radial half of the ring fingers (p. 84).

Treatment: A positive effort should be made to exclude compression of the median nerve in the carpal tunnel and, if such lesion is found, it should be treated early. Otherwise, general therapeutic principles apply (see p. 99), including muscle stimulation.

---

flexion of the hand, flexion of the thumb and index and middle fingers and extension of the index and middle fingers at the distal phalangeal joints. **(Top and middle right)** Sensory innervation of median nerve. **(Bottom right)** Position of hand in median palsy ("oath hand").

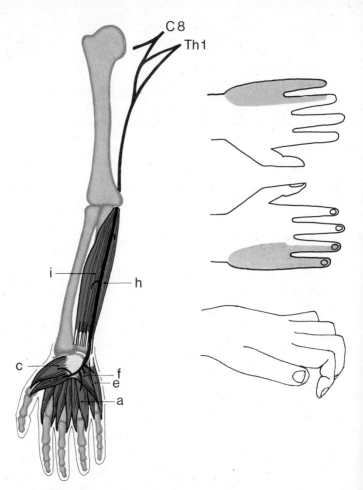

Fig. 38.—The ulnar nerve arises from the C8–T1 nerve roots of the brachial plexus and supplies: (a) interosseus muscles, 3d and 4th lumbrical muscles, (c) adductor pollicis, part of flexor pollicis brevis, (e) abductor digiti minimi, (f) opponens digiti minimi, palmaris brevis and (h) flexor carpi ulnaris (and [i] half of flexor digitorum profundus). Paralysis prevents palmar and ulnar flexion of the hand, adduction and flexion of the thumb, both adduction and

Ulnar Nerve (C8–T1)

Etiology: Compression paralysis (chess playing and occupational injury to the elbow) of the nerve in the olecranon groove: the nerve is said to ride on the tip of the medial humeral epicondyle. The main causes of ulnar palsy are fractures of the elbow, puncture wounds and pressure at the wrist. The ulnar nerve is the most commonly injured nerve in the body.

Clinical: The following muscles are paralyzed: interossei I–IV, lumbricals III and IV, adductor pollicis, flexor pollicis brevis, flexor digiti minimi, abductor digiti minimi, opponens digiti minimi and palmaris brevis. Sensory changes usually are detected over the ulnar side of the hand, including both the palmar and dorsal surfaces of the entire little finger and the medial aspect of the ring finger (p. 86). Nerve damage at the elbow produces a paralysis of the flexor carpi ulnaris and the ulnar part of flexor digitorum profundus.

Hyperextension of the fingers, especially the ring and little fingers, at the metacarpophalangeal joints combined with flexion of the middle and terminal joints produces the deformity of *"clawhand."* The interosseous muscles and adductor pollicis are visibly atrophic; the hypothenar eminence is flattened; the metacarpophalangeal joint of the thumb remains hyperextended. In order to grip a sheet of paper between his thumb and index finger, the patient utilizes flexor pollicis longus (because adductor pollicis is paralyzed); consequently, the terminal interphalangeal joint of the thumb is flexed, not extended, during the movement *(Froment's sign).*

Differential diagnosis: The most important entities to exclude are syringomyelia (often Horner's syndrome is present and other clinical levels are affected), C8–T1 nerve root damage (segmental sensory disturbances over the upper arm as well) and progressive spinal muscular atrophy (no sensory abnormality).

Treatment: Physiotherapy and electrical stimulation (see p. 99).

---

abduction of all four fingers, flexion of the ring and little fingers at the metacarpophalangeal joints and extension of the terminal interphalangeal joints. (Note: some muscles not shown—see text.) Top and middle line drawings: cutaneous innervation of ulnar nerve. Bottom line drawing: position of hand in ulnar palsy. "clawhand."

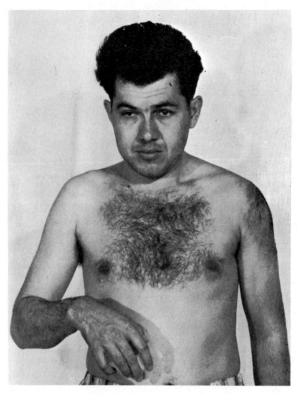

Fig. 39.—Lesion of the C8–T1 segments with Horner's syndrome (pinpoint pupil, ptosis and enophthalmos), paralysis and atrophy of the small muscles of the hand and sensory loss over the fingers (not the thumb) and ulnar forearm. The picture corresponds to a lower brachial plexus palsy, the Dejerine-Klumpke type of paralysis. The patient illustrated suffered from syringomyelia involving the anterior horn cells. C7 was involved also, resulting in weakness of wrist extension.

Upper Brachial Plexus (Erb's) Palsy (C4–6)

Etiology: The main causes are excessive stretching, compression (general anesthesia, carrying heavy weights), infiltrating tumors (apex of lung, carcinoma or pleural endothelioma—*Pancoast's syndrome*), arterial aneurysms and stab or gunshot wounds. *Avulsion* of one or more *nerve roots* (ski or motorcycle injuries) produces a similar clinical picture.

Clinical: The following muscles are paralyzed: biceps, brachialis, brachioradialis and supinator and, less often, the supra- and infraspinatus, serratus anterior and teres minor. Sensory changes are present over the outer aspect of the shoulder and upper arm, sometimes also over the radial side of the forearm. The biceps reflex is absent whereas the triceps reflex remains intact.

Lower Brachial Plexus (Dejerine-Klumpke's) Palsy (C7–T1)

Etiology: Birth trauma and (much less frequently) following injury in later life.

Clinical: Paralysis of the long and short finger flexors, sometimes also the wrist flexors. The long extensors and triceps muscle usually are spared. A clawhand develops. Damage to the sympathetic nerve supply to the eye (via C8 and T1) on the affected side is reflected in an ipsilateral miosis, ptosis and enophthalmos. Sensory changes are confined to the ulnar side of the forearm and hand.

Cervical Root Syndrome (see also Lateral Disk Prolapse, p. 91)

The most common is the *C7 syndrome:* pain radiates down the arm into the index, middle and ring fingers. This area of the skin is hypalgesic and there is a similar band over the palm of the hand, the forearm and the outer aspect of the upper arm. Triceps and pronator teres are weak and the triceps reflex is diminished. Both triceps and thenar muscles are atrophic. The *C8 syndrome* involves the ring and middle fingers: the triceps brachii, hypothenar muscles and interossei are atrophic.

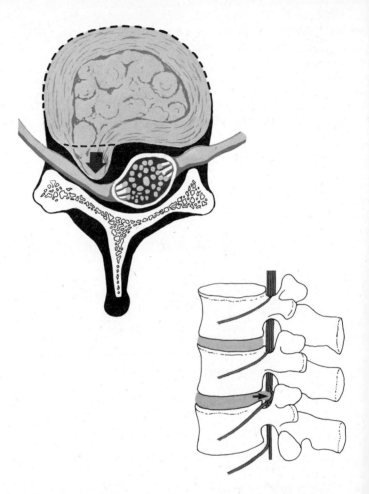

Fig. 40.—Semidiagrammatic representation of lateral lumbar disk prolapse, viewed from above **(top)** and the side **(bottom).** The adjacent ipsilateral nerve root is compressed, causing segmental sensory and motor deficits. Prolapse of the L4–5 disk leads to an L5 lesion, L5–S1 prolapse to an S1 lesion. Reflex muscle spasm, interruption of the reflex arc and pain on stretching the affected nerve root are additional findings.

Lateral Disk Prolapse (Nerve Root Syndrome)

Etiology: Clinically severe mechanical stress on the intervertebral disk apparatus in middle or advanced age (lifting heavy weights,
bending) may cause sudden lateral prolapse of part of the nucleus
pulposus. Compression of the sensory and motor nerve roots in the
intervertebral foramen leads to sensory, trophic and motor lesions
in the corresponding segment. The reflex arc is interrupted. The lumbosacral disk (L5–S) is most commonly involved, resulting in a S1
root syndrome; then L4–5 (L5 syndrome) and the lower cervical
disk spaces (C7 and C8 syndromes) see also pp. 184 and 185).

Clinical: In the L5 and S1 syndromes, stretching of the sciatic
nerve produces acute pain. It may be so severe that, with the patient supine, the leg can be raised only slightly (Lasegue's sign).
Nerve-stretch pain may even be present in the other leg (crossed
Lasegue). The patient may be unwilling to cough, sneeze or strain
(defecation) for fear that the resulting increase in cerebrospinal fluid
pressure will produce further root pain. In the *L5 syndrome*, a band
of hypesthesia is present over the lateral side of the shin, radiating
into the great toe. A characteristic deficit is an isolated paralysis of
the extensor of the great toe, and foot elevation may be weak. Muscle atrophy and loss of the posterior tibial reflex soon follow. In the
S1 syndrome, the hypesthetic band lies along the posterior surface
of the ankle and the outer side of the foot involving the 3d–5th toes.
The patient is unable to stand on his toes, and the ankle jerk is impaired. Foot pronation is weak. Leg flexors and the gluteal muscles
may be involved also. Muscle atrophy follows.

Treatment: In cases of weakness or paralysis or prolonged
pain, operation. Conservative management—bed rest, analgesics
and steroids may be successful.

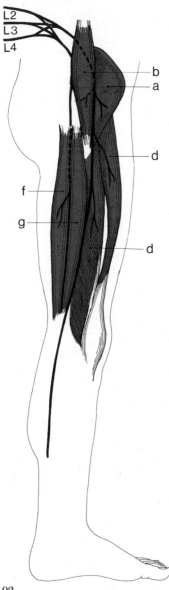

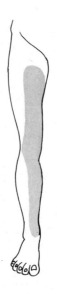

FIG. 41.—The obturator nerve (L2–4) supplies the following muscles: pectineus, obturator externus, adductors minimus, brevis, longus *(g)* and magnus, as well as gracilis *(f)*. Paralysis prevents adduction (and hinders external rotation). The femoral nerve (L2–4) supplies the following muscles: *(a* and *b)* iliopsoas, sartorius and *(d)* quadriceps femoris. Paralysis prevents knee extension and hip flexion; external rotation and flexion of the knee are impaired slightly.

Obturator Nerve (L2-4)

Etiology: Very rarely in fractures of the pelvis, obturator hernias.

Clinical: Paralysis of the adductor muscles, which is obvious during walking. Sensory loss over medial and distal aspects of thigh.

Femoral Nerve (L2-4) (see also p. 184)

Etiology: May be damaged in herniorraphy, retroperitoneal lymphoma, psoas hematoma (anticoagulants, hemophilia), after overstretching of the hip joint and other trauma.

Clinical: If the femoral nerve is severely damaged, the iliopsoas muscle will be weak; thus, hip movements are impaired. Paralysis of the sartorius (flexor and external rotator), pectineus (adductor) and the adductor muscles (partial innervation) is relatively unimportant, but paralysis of the quadriceps femoris prevents the patient from extending his leg at the knee. The knee jerk is absent. Sensory changes are present over the anterior thigh and the medial aspect of the calf (saphenous nerve).

Treatment: Remedial exercises, muscle stimulation.

Lateral Femoral Cutaneous Nerve (L2-3) (see also p. 184)

Etiology: This purely sensory nerve may be damaged at its point of exit from the pelvis. According to Mumenthaler, an "inguinal ligament syndrome" exists: the nerve makes an angle of nearly 90 degress in its passage through the tendinous fibers of the oblique abdominal muscles; consequently, it is damaged easily. Predisposing causes are pregnancy, wearing a tight corset, a pendulous abdomen, a strenuous march or prolonged recumbency with a leg outstretched.

Clinical: The sensory deficit involves the entire outer aspect of the thigh and commonly is associated with pain and paresthesias. This variety of *meralgia paresthetica* is particularly long lasting. Neurolysis may bring relief.

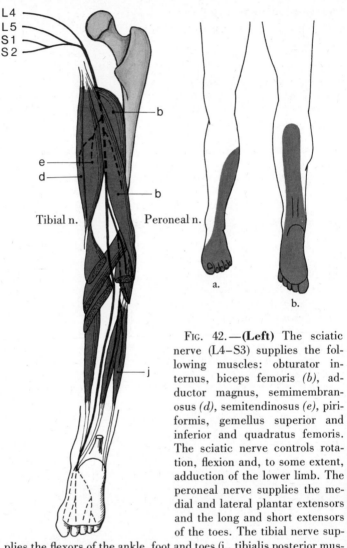

FIG. 42.—**(Left)** The sciatic nerve (L4–S3) supplies the following muscles: obturator internus, biceps femoris *(b)*, adductor magnus, semimembranosus *(d)*, semitendinosus *(e)*, piriformis, gemellus superior and inferior and quadratus femoris. The sciatic nerve controls rotation, flexion and, to some extent, adduction of the lower limb. The peroneal nerve supplies the medial and lateral plantar extensors and the long and short extensors of the toes. The tibial nerve supplies the flexors of the ankle, foot and toes (j., tibialis posterior muscle). **(Right)** Sensory impairment with *(a)* common peroneal palsy and *(b)* tibial nerve palsy.

94

Sciatic Nerve (L4–S3) (see also p. 185)

Etiology: Damage to this nerve, the longest and largest peripheral nerve in the body, complicates fracture dislocations, inexpertly administrated *injections* into the gluteal muscles, stretching, etc.

Clinical: Most frequently damaged is the trunk of the peroneal nerve, which is discussed separately. Paralysis of the knee flexors (biceps femoris, semimembranosus and semitendinosus) and adductor magnus follows with partial weakness of adduction. The tibial nerve also may be damaged, impairing plantar flexion of the foot. The patient is unable to rise on his toes, and adduction and supination of the foot are restricted. The toes cannot be extended at the metatarsophalangeal or interphalangeal joints. Talipes calcaneus and talipes cavus result. Sensation is impaired over the posterior surface of the ankle and the sole of the foot.

Peroneal Nerve, Sciatic Trunk (L4–S2) (see also p. 184)

Etiology: Damage to this nerve is quite common. Immediately after its origin from the sciatic, the peroneal nerve winds around the head of the fibula and separates into superficial and deep branches. It may be damaged by simple movements such as crossing the legs, pressure from an ineptly applied plaster cast, overstretching from prolonged kneeling or crouching ("turnip planter's palsy") or "spontaneously" in unconscious patients.

Clinical: The superficial peroneal nerve supplies the peroneal muscles (weakness of the ankle dorsiflexors) and mediates sensation over the lateral aspect of the ankle and dorsum of the foot. Injury of the deep peroneal nerve results in paralysis of ankle and toe dorsiflexion ("stepping gait"). The patient is unable to stand on his heels. The deep peroneal has a cutaneous twig supplying the skin over the base of the great and second toes. Prolonged chronaxy and muscle atrophy are poor prognostic signs.

Differential Diagnosis of Neurogenic Bladder Disturbances

Name	Signs	Level of Lesion
Uncontrolled bladder	Uncontrollable emptying—no residual urine—active emptying possible	Cortex of paracentral lobule or cortico-spinal tracts
Automatic bladder	Reflex emptying—can be triggered. Very little residual urine	Spinal cord lesions, sacral centers intact
Motor atonic bladder	Bladder muscle relaxed. Spastic sphincter. Voluntary emptying impossible. Retention with overflow	Damage of anterior (or lateral) horn cells or anterior spinal nerve roots—the motor half of the bladder reflex arc
Sensory atonic bladder	Deafferentation. No urge to micturate. Retention with overflow	Posterior nerve root and/or "posterior horn" damage—the sensory half of the bladder reflex arc
Autonomic bladder	Flaccid bladder with overflow; later, slight local contractions leading to shrinkage with bladder wall hypertrophy; no voluntary control	Injury of bladder center in the conus medullaris—sensory (afferent) or motor (efferent) segments of reflex arc

The *spinal center* is S2–4. The parasympathetic *efferent fibers* pass in the S2–4 roots and the nervi erigentes to the detrusor and internal sphincter muscles. *Motor efferents* also pass in the S2–4 roots and the pudendal nerve to the external sphincter muscle.

Sensory afferent fibers pass in the hypogastric, pelvic and pudendal nerves.

Damage to Lumbar Plexus (L1–4)

The most common cause is metastatic disease of the pelvis involving especially the pelvic lymph nodes, and extensive x-irradiation. The hip flexors and rotators are paralyzed and adduction and extension of the thigh is impossible. The adductor reflex and knee jerk are absent. Sensation is impaired over the inguinal region (iliohypogastric nerve) and scrotum (labium) (genitofemoral and ilioinguinal nerves), over the posterior (posterior femoral cutaneous nerve) and lateral (lateral femoral cutaneous nerve) thigh.

Complete paralysis is rare (see also pp. 184 and 185).

Damage to sacral plexus (L5–S3)

Metastases of pelvic cancer (uterus or prostate) are the most common causes. The deficits correspond roughly to sciatic nerve damage.

Damage to Pudendal Plexus (S2–4)

Nerves from this plexus supply the perineal region (perineal and posterior scrotal nerves) and the genitalia (dorsal clitoral nerve). These nerves carry the important sympathetic and parasympathetic innervation of the bladder and rectal muscles. Extensive damage leads to loss of sphincter tone and consequent disturbances of bladder emptying. If only the sensory pathway is interrupted ("deafferentated bladder"), the bladder ceases to contract reflexly and retention with overflow occurs. If only the motor pathway is interrupted ("de-efferentated bladder"), the bladder similarly is paralyzed and retention with overflow results ("denervated bladder"). If both segments of the reflex arc are affected, the bladder is initially flaccid and distensible but contracts later. Differentiation from a cauda equina syndrome may be difficult or impossible.

Peripheral Nerve Injuries

Time Scale of Healing (according to Foerster)

	Shortest	Average	Longest
Radial nerve	6	25	40 months
Median nerve	4	19	31 months
Ulnar nerve	4	18	31 months
Sciatic nerve	4	25	40 months
Peroneal nerve	11	23	36 months

Percentage Reduction of Work Capacity in Peripheral Nerve Lesions

Oculomotor nerve	10–30%	
Trochlear nerve	10–20%	
Abducent nerve	10–20%	

	Right	Left
Axillary nerve	30%	20%
Long thoracic nerve	20%	20%
Musculocutaneous nerve	25%	20%
Radial nerve, upper	35%	30%
middle	30%	25%
lower	20%	15%
Ulnar nerve, middle	25%	20%
lower	20%	15%
Median nerve, middle	35%	30%
lower	30%	25%
Median + ulnar nerves	60%	50%
Radial + median nerves	60%	50%
Ulnar + radial nerves	50%	40%
Brachial plexus—Erb's palsy	30%	25%
—Klumpke	75%	60%
—Total	75%	66²/₃%
Sciatic nerve, upper	50%	50%
lower	40%	40%
Femoral nerve, upper	40%	40%
lower	30%	30%

Peroneal nerve, common	25%	25%
superficial division	10%	10%
deep division	25%	25%
Tibial nerve	30%	30%

Percentages apply to a right-handed subject; vice versa if left-handed.

GENERAL PRINCIPLES OF MANAGEMENT OF PERIPHERAL NERVE INJURIES (ROOT AND PLEXUS DAMAGE)

Whenever possible, specific treatment should be instituted. The following general rules apply: essential to prevent *nursing complications* —faulty positioning of the limbs may lead to contractures and a fixed position leads to destructive obliteration of joints. Inadequate nursing attention is responsible for bedsores. The carelss use of heat may cause burns, which the patient is initially unable to feel immediately. In completely paralyzed extremities, the absence of muscular activity poses the threat of local circulatory impairment (stasis), which may be complicated in severe polyneuritides by deep vein thrombosis or fatal embolism. Essential and regular physiotherapy, the use of a bed cradle to keep the weight of the bedclothes off the feet, appropiate splinting of paralyzed upper limbs (to prevent joint capsule adhesions due to the weight of the paralyzed arm) and meticulous nursing care of the skin.

Denervated muscles atrophy rapidly. Provided only that some activity remains present in one or more muscles, appropriate active exercises are permissible to prevent further *muscle atrophy*. Regular passive movements are necessary in paralyzed patients to preserve mobility of the joints. Electrotherapy is indicated: each paralyzed muscle should be stimulated electrically repeatedly, daily if possible, to forestall the development of atrophy. At the first sign of reappearance of active movement, planned exercises should be initiated to exploit them and to utilize the patient's initially primitive efforts in rebuilding more sophisticated function.

The results of treatment reflect directly the dedication of nursing personnel, the optimal utilization of the physiotherapy department, the personal involvement of the patient and the use of electrotherapy. This is also true following nerve suture or nerve entrapment surgery.

99

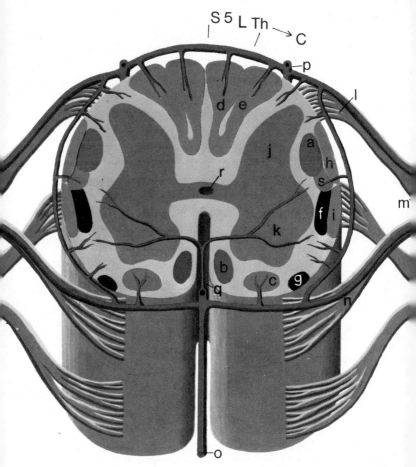

FIG. 43.—Cross section of spinal cord (diagrammatic). *(a)* Lateral corticospinal tract. *(b)* Anterior corticospinal tract. *(c)* Extrapyramidal tracts. *(d* and *e)* Posterior (sensory) columns. *(f* and *g)* Lateral and anterior spinothalamic tracts. *(h* and *i)* Posterior and anterior spinocerebellar tracts. *(j)* Posterior horn. *(k)* Anterior horn. *(l)* Posterior root. *(m)* Spinal ganglion. *(n)* Anterior root. *(o)* Anterior spinal artery. *(p)* Posterior spinal artery. *(q)* Anterior longitudinal fissure. *(r)* Central canal. *(s)* Rubrospinal tract.

Spinal Cord Diseases

The clinical features of spinal cord lesions depend largely on their level. Several diseases affect predominantly or almost exclusively the ganglion cells (anterior poliomyelitis = disease of the anterior horn cells; herpes zoster = a disease of the dorsal root ganglia), spinal tracts (tabes dorsalis = posterior column lesion; Friedreich's ataxia = a lesion predominantly involving the spinocerebellar tracts; familial spastic paraplegia = diseases of the pyramidal tracts) or specific arterial territories. Other diseases (myelitis, spinal cord trauma, intraspinal tumors) may produce a transverse myelopathy; some injuries lead to the Brown-Seguard syndrome. Syringomyelia is most likely to damage the parts of the spinal cord around the central canal. Very similar symptoms may be present in gliomas of the spinal cord.

Circulatory disturbances produce additional symptoms in patients with tumors and inflammatory lesions. A detailed knowledge of spinal cord anatomy, therefore, is a prerequisite for evaluating function. Careful neurologic examination remains a particularly important part of the total examination of such a patient. Observant patients are able, in the course of history taking, to contribute significantly to the diagnosis. *CSF examination* usually is unavoidable (to diagnose infectious diseases and to exclude narrowing or obstruction of the CSF pathways: *Queckenstedt's sign*, sequestered CSF with a very high protein content). Sometimes electromyography contributes to the diagnosis by revealing signs of spinal denervation. If a tumor is suspected, myelography is essential. A sweat test may help to localize the lesion.

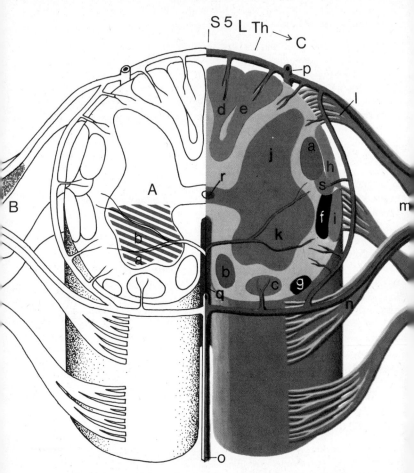

FIG. 44.—Location of the most severe spinal cord changes in anterior poliomyelitis (*A*, diagonal hatching) and herpes zoster (*B*, shaded area). In poliomyelitis, the anterior horn contains degenerate cells and phagocytes (neurophagia) and, later, microglia (rod cells). The spinal cord initially is hyperemic and swollen at this level. In herpes zoster, the spinal ganglion is swollen and shows lymphocytic and plasma cell infiltration, vacuolated ganglion cells, hemorrhagic necrosis and pericytic proliferation.

ANTERIOR POLIOMYELITIS

Etiology: This infection of the anterior horns is caused by viruses (type I = Brunhilde strain, type II = Lansing strain, type III = Leon strain). It may appear as an epidemic illness in the summer months in circumstances of poor hygiene and filth, not merely as a paralysis of childhood (old name = infantile paralysis). The incubation period of 4–12 days is followed by prodromal enteritic or catarrhal stage and some days later, in 1–2%, by involvement of the anterior horn cells. After a fluctuating meningitic stage, the appropriate muscles become weak or paralyzed.

Clinical: The picture is dominated by paralysis, especially of the trunk muscles, which follows hours or days after a febrile illness. Life is threatened by paralysis of the respiratory muscles and is endangered by paralysis of the pharyngeal muscles (swallowing). After some weeks, an incomplete recovery usually occurs. Permanent deficits include significant muscular atrophy, secondary circulatory disturbances and bone and joint deformities. Initially, the rheobase is slight reduced and then increased and the chronaxy is increased. The EMG usually shows positive sharp waves and signs of denervation. Late complications in children are scoliosis and an atrophic limb.

Diagnosis: In the early stages, differential diagnosis from polyneuritis is aided by determining the level of neutralizing antibodies and isolating the causal organism from faucial washings and feces, also CSF examination (100–1,000/3 cells, initially polymorphonuclear cells and later lymphocytes and a slight protein increase).

Treatment: Prophylaxis is accomplished through the use of inactivated virus, either orally (Sabin) or by injection (Salk). Carelessness concerning inoculation threatens a return of this already rare disease! Tracheostomy and positive-pressure respiration are required in respiratory paralysis and a permanently indwelling gastric tube is necessary in paralytic dysphagia. Prevention of bedsores, electrical stimulation and physiotherapy of the paralyzed muscles. Early orthopedic advice about deformities!

HERPES ZOSTER

This viral disease of the spinal ganglia is characterized by a skin eruption, pain and sensory loss in the appropriate dermatomal segment. Rarely, meningitis or myelitis may accompany it.

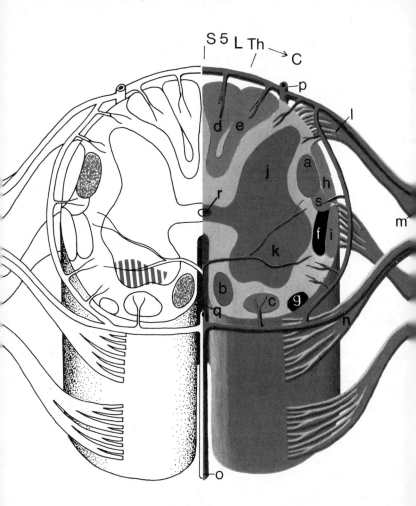

Fig. 45.—In familial spastic paraplegia, a grayish yellow discoloration and shrinkage of the pyramidal tracts is present. Fatty degeneration is followed by glial scarring and degeneration of the axis cylinders. In spinal muscular atrophy, the anterior horn cells degenerate and the anterior roots become atrophic. In amyotrophic lateral sclerosis, both upper and lower motor neurons show degenerative changes.

FAMILIAL SPASTIC PARAPLEGIA

Etiology: Atrophy of the pyramidal cells in the 3rd and 5th cortical layers of the precentral gyrus leads to degeneration of the corticospinal tracts—rare; dominant hereditary disease.

Clinical: The picture of muscle weakness, spasticity and increased reflexes usually is observed in middle age (rare in childhood and old age). A Friedreich's foot and pseudobulbar palsy may be additional signs.

SPINAL MUSCULAR ATROPHY

Etiology: Selective ganglion cell degeneration of the anterior horns and motor cranial nerve nuclei leads to atrophy of motor units and muscles. One variety *(Werdnig-Hoffman)*, an autosomal recessive disease of early infancy, tends to involve all voluntary muscles, sparing ocular muscles; another *(Kugelberg-Welander)*, also inherited in autosomal recessive fashion, affects the pelvic muscles of older children; the adult variety *(Duchenne-Aran)*, which exhibits no recognizable heritable pattern, commences in the distal muscles of the arms. The *Vulpian-Bernhardt* variety is circumscribed in the extent of muscle involvement, usually being confined to the shoulder girdle. The early childhood variety has a rapid course; the other forms may be only slowly progressive. *Bulbar palsy* (speech and swallowing disturbances) is a threat to life.

Clinical: Muscle paralysis, atrophy, fasciculations and absent reflexes (interrupted reflex arc) without sensory symptoms should prompt suspicion of the diagnosis. Signs of denervation in the EMG, and a group atrophy of muscle fibers on biopsy, confirm the diagnosis.

Treatment: Isometric muscle retraining.

MOTOR NEURON DISEASE (see also p. 14) (Amyotrophic Lateral Sclerosis)

Motor neuron disease represents, to a certain extent, a combination of the preceeding two diseases, yet it possesses its own identity. Affected persons usually are over 45 years of age. The upper and lower motor neurons (pyramidal tract and anterior horns) are affected. The etiology is not certain. Symptomatic varieties can be excluded.

Clinical: The triad of spasticity, muscular atrophy and spontaneous fasciculations is present. The diagnosis is confirmed by EMG and muscle biopsy, as in spinal muscular atrophy. Because of its progressive course, the disease seldom extends over 3 years and terminates, with aspiration pneumonia and asphyxia, in death.

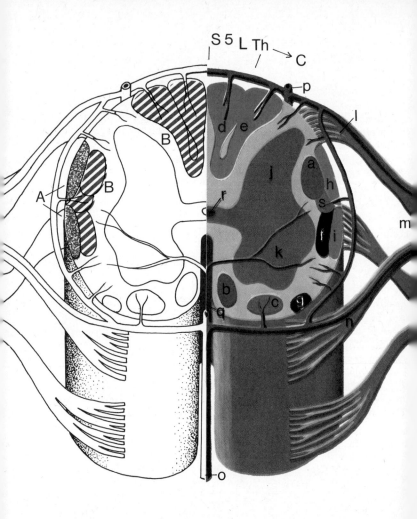

Fig. 46.—The heredoataxias involve the spinocerebellar system *(A)* preferentially (but not exclusively). In addition, posterior column degeneration and, later, a severe gliosis occur. Subacute combined system disease results in focal spongy degeneration of posterior and lateral columns of the spinal cord.

Spinocerebellar Diseases (Heredoataxias)

Etiology: Friedreich's ataxia is recessive, *Roussy-Lévy syndrome* is dominant. Degeneration of the spinocerebellar tracts, the corticospinal tracts and posterior columns occurs. In the Roussy-Lévy variety, a peroneal muscular atrophy and tremor appears. Associations are described with hypogonadism, degeneration of retinal pigment, etc.; many families exhibit characteristic combinations of symptoms among their affected members.

Clinical: Presenting features are ataxia, sometimes to a striking degree, absent position sense, pes cavus with hammer toes ("Friedreich's foot"), absent reflexes, reduced muscle tone, Babinski's sign and dysarthria. The disease begins about the 15th year and the patient is usually bedridden within a decade. Gait and hand movements are severely restricted; the patient's handwriting is grossly abnormal (hyper- and dysmetric): megalographia.

Treatment: Physiotherapy. No specific treatment is known.

Combined Systems Disease

Etiology: Inadequate vitamin B_{12} (cyanocobalamin) absorption, due to a deficiency of gastric intrinsic factor, is the main cause. Patchy degeneration of myelin sheaths occurs and, later, of the axis cylinders: focal areas become confluent, particularly in the pyramidal tracts and posterior columns of the cervical and thoracic spinal cord. The brain and peripheral nerves may also be affected.

Clinical: Paresthesias and sensory disturbances (diminished vibration sense) appear first. Later, ataxia, pyramidal tract signs, spasticity and disturbances of bladder and rectal function follow. Psychoses and other mental changes may occur. The clinical deficits usually are most obvious distally.

Diagnosis: Every third patient has no evidence of pernicious anemia, but a histamine-resistant achlorhydria is often present. The *Schilling test* confirms the diagnosis: at least 10% of radioactive vitamin B_{12} administered orally is absorbed and excreted in the urine. If intrinsic factor alone is deficient, absorption and urinary excretion returns to normal if exogenous intrinsic factor is added to the radioactive vitamin B_{12} dose.

Treatment: Intramuscular injections of vitamin B_{12}, 1,000 gm twice weekly. Physiotherpay.

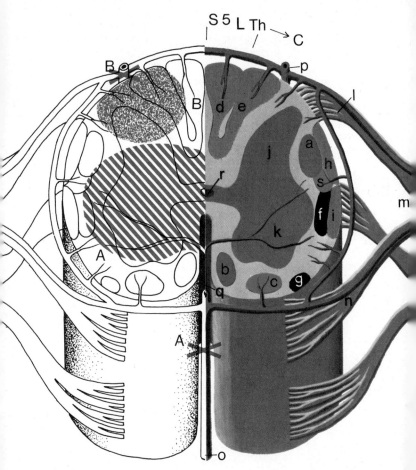

FIG. 47.—Arteriolar disease, less commonly atherosclerosis, threatens the circulation of the spinal cord of elderly subjects. Occlusive lesions at various sites or reduced perfusion of a specific artery at a distance leads to characteristic syndromes: the anterior spinal artery (A) syndrome is associated with infarction of the anterior and medial portions of the spinal cord, the posterior spinal artery (B) syndrome with lesions of the posterior horn and posterior columns.

108

About 5% of the vascular lesions of the CNS affect the spinal cord. Usually arteriosclerosis is present. Arterial disturbances may be classified schematically into several syndromes, depending on the vascular territory predominantly affected. The *anterior spinal artery syndrome* affects parts of the anterior horns, anterolateral columns and anterior parts of the pyramidal tracts. The paralysis first is flaccid; then a spactic para- (or tetra-) paresis, a dissociated sensory anesthesia below the level of the infarct and bladder and rectal disturbances occur. Fibrillation may be visible at the level of the anterior horn lesion and, later, atrophy occurs. There is moderate recovery over a period of months. *Syndrome of the great radicular artery of Adamkiewicz* = sudden and complete sensorimotor paraplegia at the lower thoracic or upper lumbar level with bladder and bowel dysfunction. Poor recovery. Later, spasticity and automatic bladder; *posterior spinal artery syndrome* = unilateral sensory changes of sudden onset and paresthesias with a tendency to moderate recovery. Weakness is exceptional. These syndromes may be intermittent, presenting as Dejerine's syndrome, i.e., *intermittent claudication* of the cord. Typically, the symptoms improve with rest and are aggravated by strenuous physical exertion (walking). However, the clinical picture may not always be so clear-cut and, in older persons, less-well-defined, apparently vascular symptoms are encountered, which progress in a stepwise, apoplectiform or chronic manner. Weakness of the legs, atrophy of the hand muscles and spastic tetraparesis are common. *Vascular myelopathy* of this type may be difficult to differentiate from motor neuron disease, apart from the obvious age difference. Subacute necrotizing myelitis (Foix-Alajouanine) is thought to have a vascular basis, viz., angiomatous malformations *(angiodysgenetic myelomalacia)*, which leads in a stepwise progression through pain, sensory disturbances and paralysis, to paraplegia.

Treatment: As for intracranial vascular lesions.

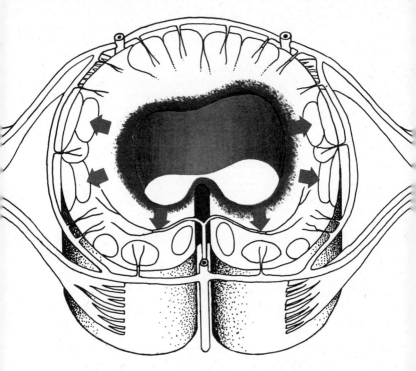

FIG. 48. —Syringomyelia is characterized by cavitation, which involves several segments in the longitudinal direction or even the whole length of the spinal cord. The cervical cord is affected most often. The cavities appear punched out and are surrounded by a narrow zone of demyelination and moderate gliosis. The cavity may be lined by ependymal cells but it does not possess an intact membrane. Fibrosis of vessels, connective tissue proliferation (see also Fig. 39).

Etiology: The tube-like cavitation in the spinal cord or medulla oblongata and the more rostral brainstem (= *syringobulbia*) occurs—commonly after minor trauma—particularly in men (2:1). A predisposing factor is spinal dysraphism. The pathologic changes, which are surrounded by glial cell degeneration, are most common in the cervical and thoracic cord. The crossed sensory tracts of the diseased segments and, later, the pyramidal tracts, lateral cerebellar tracts and anterior horns are all involved.

Clinical: The presenting sign often is pain—posterior horn, funicular or quadrantic in type. The typical picture is one of segmental *dissociated sensory disturbances* occurring in a subject 20–30 years of age (but also earlier or later), followed by a flaccid paralysis of the affected segment, absent reflexes, muscle atrophy and EMG evidence of denervation. Later, contralateral dissociated sensory disturbances below the level of the lesion and an ipsilateral spastic paralysis develop. Further sensory changes are rare. Secondary complications include autonomic disturbances, joint changes and spinal deformity. In lesions of the cervical cord, *Horner's syndrome* is common: ipsilateral ptosis, miosis and enophthalmos. Typical lesions are numerous scars on the fingers, toes and extremities due to skin wounds that have healed poorly— the patient appreciates burns or cuts as tactile sensations only, since pain sensation is lost. The patient's attention first may be drawn to the skin burn through the unpleasant smell of burning flesh. A profusely scarred atrophic *"ape hand"* prompts a spot diagnosis of syringomyelia.

Diagnosis: Intramedullary gliomas may be extremely difficult to distinguish from syringomyelia; both conditions are slowly progressive and may exhibit the same signs and symptoms. The clinical course of syringomyelia spans decades.

Treatment: There is no convincing evidence that either radiotherapy or surgical ablation of the cavities exerts any beneficial effect on the disease, nor that measures to improve the circulation are helpful. No medical treatment. Physiotherapy.

Intraspinal Tumors (Glioma, Glioblastoma)

Symptoms similar to syringomyelia. Operation often unsuccessful. "Descending" motor and sensory deficits.

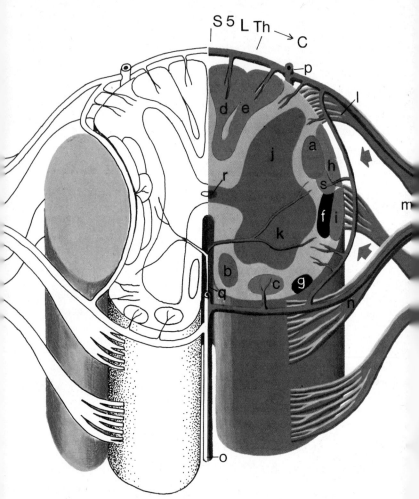

Fig. 49.—Extraspinal (extramedullary) tumors may be intradural or epidural. The diagram illustrates an intradural tumor, of which the most common type by far is a meningioma. Neurinomas are slightly less frequent followed by arteriovenous malformations, plaques of adhesive arachnoiditis, ependymomas and teratomas. The well-defined tumor compresses the spinal cord against the opposite wall of the vertebral canal. Central pain and contralateral symptoms may be the presenting features.

Intra- and epidural tumors possess great practical importance because they may be operable. The epidural tumors arise mostly from bone, i.e., the surrounding vertebrae: metastatic cancer is the most common, then sarcoma, hemangioma or abscess; spinal tuberculosis (Pott's disease) and giant cell tumors are less frequent. Intradural tumors in the thoracic cord are meningiomas; elsewhere, neurinomas are most common; hemangiomas are less common.

Clinical: The end stage, viz., a complete transverse myelopathy with spastic paraplegia, sensory loss and rectal and bladder dysfunction, must be prevented at all costs. Early symptoms are radicular pain and segmental sensory disturbances; these are followed by uni- or bilateral distal weakness, increased reflexes, Babinski's sign and increased muscle tone. The patient experiences difficulty emptying his bladder; he may be surprised to find that bladder emptying suddenly becomes automatic and that he cannot reach the toilet in time. Dull back pain may be experienced at the level of the lesion. Progression after months or years; the level of muscle weakness and the sensory loss may ascend. Segmental muscle atrophy, also, may occur at the level of the lesion.

Diagnosis: The fully developed clinical picture is typical. Important in early diagnosis is lumbar puncture (nearly always: raised protein) and a *positive Queckenstedt sign*, which is made more definite by simultaneous lumbar and suboccipital testing. The diagnosis is confirmed by myelography (oil = Pantopaque; newer water-soluble contrast media = Amipaque), which outlines the tumor. Roentgenograms of the spine and chest are essential: they may reveal focal bone destruction or widening of the spinal canal, enlargement of an intervertebral foramen in neurinoma or rib, vertebral or pulmonary metastases.

Treatment: Evidence of metastatic deposits is no contraindication to immediate neurosurgical decompression and removal of the tumor. Complete cure may be possible. Postoperative physiotherapy is particularly important.

Recognition and Treatment of Acute Paraplegic Syndromes

History: Initially, the patient may complain only of the legs giving way or of difficulty climbing stairs and sensory changes in the lower limbs. Bladder emptying takes longer and requires manual pressure. Constipation. Later: complete paralysis. Details of the backache are important for determining the level. The patient is often indifferent and euphoric.

Physical Findings: Reduced or absent sensation below a specific dermatome. There may be a narrow band of hyperesthesia, 1–2 segments wide above the level of the lesion, and the two vertebrae immediately above are painful to percussion. Usually a flaccid paralysis is present initially, later spastic. In lesions above the lower thoracic cord, Babinski's and Rossolimo's signs are present with increasing frequency. Urinary retention (residual urine) and constipation.

Investigations: Roentgenograms of the whole spine to exclude tuberculosis (Pott's disease) or the spine, hemangioma of bone, metastases or spinal osteomyelitis. Chest roentgenogram to exclude bronchial carcinoma or metastases.

CSF: Pandy's reaction to identify increased protein. Cell count to demonstrate inflammatory lesion (myelitis, neurosyphilis, tuberculosis, sarcoidosis, etc.). Queckenstedt's test: if the CSF pressure rises on abdominal pressure yet fails to do so on jugular compression, the presence of a space-occupying lesion of the spinal cord can be assumed. (If in doubt, simultaneous cisternal and lumbar pressure readings.) Pantopaque myelography with AP and lateral roentgenograms will accurately demonstrate the level of the tumor.

Treatment: Proved space-occupying lesions (tumors, hematomas, central disk protrusions) require operation on the same day. Also: anti-inflammatory and anti-edema measures, circulatory support.

114

Central Disk Protrusion (Prolapse)

A central prolapse of an intervertebral disk that compresses the spinal cord may occur suddenly, usually after mechanical strain. This condition should be considered in any bilateral cord syndrome with a transverse lesion (paresis to paraplegia, sensory impairment and bladder and bowel disturbances). Lumbar central disk prolapse causes a *cauda equina syndrome* with root pain in both legs, *saddle anesthesia* and retention of urine.

Diagnosis: If a central disk prolapse is suspected, the diagnosis should be verified as quickly as possible by lumbar puncture, Queckenstedt's test and myelography. A golden rule should be observed: that operation must follow immediately—"before the sun goes down"—if severe, irreversible deficits are to be avoided.

Spinal Cord Trauma

Trauma of the spinal cord with or without vertebral fracture-dislocations may cause any type of cord syndrome, including a complete transverse myelopathy. Direct pressure effects of fractured vertebrae, *epidural hematomas,* whiplash injuries (spinal cord contusion) and circulatory disturbances interfere with the blood supply; injuring a segmental radicular artery leads to cord damage. The initial symptoms during the first few days are the result of a combination of effects—hematoma formation and traumatic edema. Within a few weeks, the flaccid paralysis becomes spastic. The reflexes usually are brisk and Babinski's sign is present. An indwelling catheter is required for the urinary retention, and special vigilance to prevent bedsores. Operative measures to decompress the spinal cord usually are unsuccessful. The most important part of management is a planned program of physiotherapy aimed at rehabilitation. *Whiplash injuries of the vertebral column* as a result of automobile accidents are seen with increasing frequency nowadays: cervical root symptoms are prominent; spinal cord involvement often is slight.

Treatment: In the acute state, control of the accompanying edema is essential. The outcome will depend largely on preventing the complications of inadequate nursing (contractures, bedsores, bladder and rectal infection). Early physiotherapy.

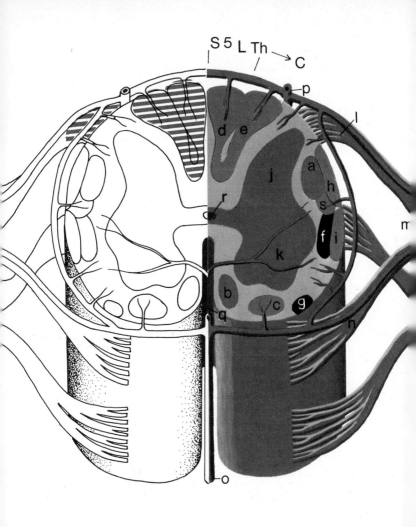

Fig. 50.—Tabes dorsalis always begins in the lumbar segments, with degeneration of the posterior nerve roots. Later, a dense gliosis develops in the dorsal columns, which become shrunken and sclerotic. The optic nerves usually are involved also. The meninges often are thickened.

116

Inflammatory Spinal Cord Diseases: Myelitis, Abscess

Myelitis usually occurs in association with inflammatory diseases of other organs or of the brain and its coverings. Of acute or sub-acute onset, it presents a clinical picture of variable severity, including complete transverse myelitis. The patient's initial complaint may be difficulty with bladder or rectal emptying or of well-localized spinal pain. The inflammatory cause is easily recognized by the raised temperature, elevated ESR, infective changes in the hemogram and disturbances of other organ systems. However, the causative microorganism may be difficult to demonstrate. Spinal cord involvement may accompany various bacterial infections: in staphylococcal infections especially, the process is likely to develop into a *spinal cord abscess*. In addition to bacterial infections, viral diseases, mycoses and protozoal and parasitic infections may affect the spinal cord. Myelitis may complicate *Behçet's disease* and the collagen vascular diseases *(systemic lumpus erythematosus, periarteritis nodosa, etc.)*.

Diagnosis: The most important step is CSF examination: the cell count depends upon the severity of the process (the more acute, the greater the proportion of polymorphonuclear leukocytes) and the nature of the microorganism. Polys are produced by bacterial infections, lymphocytes by viruses, eosinophils by parasites; plasma cells appear in spinal cord abscess and histiocytes and macrophages (lipophages) during the repair stage. The cell count never is under 100, often over 1000 mm^3. Occasionally, microorganisms may be present in the CSF. Signs of obstruction (Queckenstedt's sign, high protein levels) in bacterial infections should prompt the suspicion of the unusual complication of spinal abscess. Epidural abscess (? tuberculosis) should be considered also.

Treatment: Antibiotics if laboratory sensitivity is proved, surgical drainage of abscess.

Tabes Dorsalis

This is a late form of syphilis affecting the posterior nerve roots and posterior columns, characterized by radicular "lancinating" pains ("tabetic crises"), ataxia, reduced muscle tone, areflexia, disturbances of gait ("lusty legs"), joint deformities and sensory changes (cold and tactile hypersensitivity). For more details, see p. 149, Neurosyphilis.

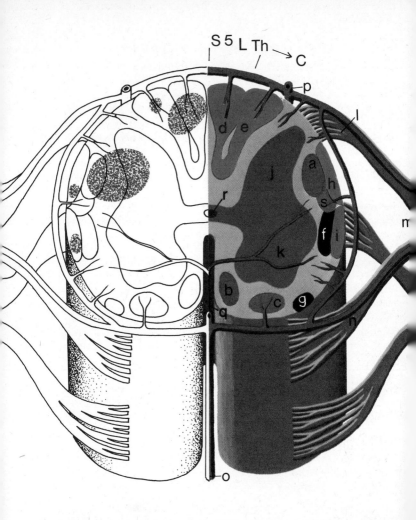

Fig. 51.—Irregular patchy degeneration of the myelin sheath, with sparing of axis cylinders and ganglion cells is typical of multiple sclerosis. Initially, an inflammatory infiltrate and demyelination are present; later, intense microgliosis and macroglial proliferation follow. The disease is multifocal, the spinal cord, pons, cerebellum and paraventricular regions are preferentially involved.

Multiple Sclerosis (Disseminated Encephalomyelitis)

Etiology: Chronic low-grade viral infection ("slow virus") and autoimmune mechanisms are postulated.

Clinical: 5–10 of every 10,000 suffer from this progressive neurologic disease—about 90% of them from recurrent attacks separated by remissions. In about 10%, the onset occurs between 16 and 21 years, in about 30% between 21 and 30. The average age at onset of the first signs is 25 to 35 years; women are affected more often. The attacks last for days to months; the average duration of the disease is 25 years. In older subjects, it may appear in a chronic progressive form. The incidence is said to be far lower in tropical climates than in Western Europe or North America. Early signs include: paresthesias and weakness of the extremities, visual disturbances and a nonspecific "pseudoneurasthenic" syndrome. According to Scheid, the completely developed picture consists of: spasticity (86.5%), cerebellar ataxia and intention tremor (58%), hypesthesia (43.3%), temporal pallor or atrophy of the optic disc (33.3%), paresthesia (33%), nystagmus (31.5%), facial palsy (31.3%), speech disturbances, particularly scanning speech (29%), external ocular palsies (26%) and bladder disturbances (20.5%). Less frequent are attacks of vertigo, paraparesis and epileptic seizures. The CSF findings may be typical, especially in the acute stage: the total protein usually is normal but the IgG fraction is elevated, a (lymphocytic) pleocytosis of $15-100$ mm^3 cells and a first-zone colloidal gold curve are present. Life is threatened by focal involvement of the vital cerebral centers (rare) or the non-neurological complications: ascending pyelonephritis, aspiration pneumonia and—rarely—decubitus sepsis.

Differential Diagnosis: Atypical patterns mimic a wide variety of intracranial and spinal cord diseases. The whole diagnostic armamentarium needs to be utilized.

Treatment: Bed rest, ACTH and physiotherapy during the attacks. Prevention of complications.

Other demyelinating encephalomyelitides also occur; some of them are para- or postinfectious, but most do not run a progressive course.

119

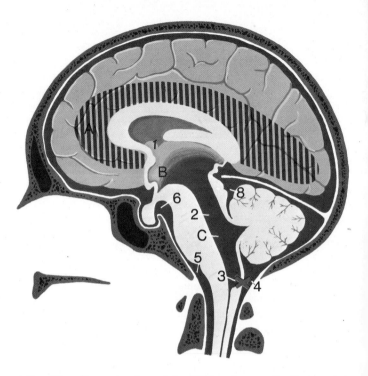

Fig. 52.—Cutaway view of the CSF pathways. Occlusion of the foramina of Magendie and Luschka (3, 4) leads to dilatation of the 4th ventricle (C), aqueduct of Sylvius (2) and the 3d (B) and lateral (A) ventricles. The result is an obstructive hydrocephalus. Occlusion of the aqueduct causes obstruction only of the 3d and lateral ventricles, and the dammed-up CSF produces pressure atrophy of the surrounding brain substance.

Cerebellar and Brain Stem Lesions

OBSTRUCTIVE HYDROCEPHALUS

Etiology: These lesions result from inflammation (arachnoiditis, ependymitis, often in early life), tumors, parasites and dysgenetic disturbances that occlude the CSF pathways and lead to ventricular enlargement. Generalized raised intracranial pressure may dramatically deteriorate the clinical picture. If the ventricles are dilated— or at least the supratentorial ventricles—one speaks of *hydrocephalus*. The following types are distinguished, in order to exclude cerebral malformations dilating the ventricles, which are associated with overproduction or impaired absorption of CSF: *dysgenetic, hypersecretory, nonresorptive (extraventricular obstructive) and obstructive hydrocephalus.*

Clinical: Congenital hydrocephalus leads to a grotesque increase in the circumference of the head: the fontanelles are larger than normal and the deep-set position of the eyeballs exposes the upper sclera (so-called setting-sun phenomenon). Mental and physical development always are delayed and the picture may lead to extensor spasms and the decerebrate state. The brain mantle may be no thicker than a few cm (CT scanning or echoencephalography will reveal it) or consist merely of a membrane that can be transilluminated (with a pocket flashlight). Percussion of the skull reveals a "crack-pot" sound. Children with less severe lesions may reach adulthood, but intellectual deficits or idiocy may be the end result. Absence of the foramen of Magendie causes a *Dandy-Walker syndrome.* This entity is a congenital defect of fusion and resembles the *Arnold-Chiari malformation,* in which a tongue-like projection of the cerebellum herniates through the foramen magnum and causes an internal hydrocephalus. The latter may be accompanied by anomalies of the *craniovertebral angle,* by cranium bifidum, spina bifida and meningo(myelo)cele.

Treatment: Early drainage by CSF shunting—ventriculocisternostomy, ventriculoatrial or ventriculoperitoneal bypass.

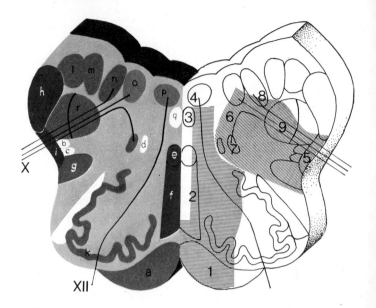

FIG. 53.—Transverse section of the medulla oblongata. *(a)* corticospinal tract, *(b)* rubrospinal tract, *(c)* reticulospinal tract, *(d)* vestibulospinal tract, *(e)* anterior spinothalamic tract, *(f)* medial lemniscus, *(g)* lateral spinothalamic tract, *(h)* inferior cerebellar peduncle, *(i)* spinocerebellar tracts, *(k)* inferior olive, *(l)* nucleus cuneatus, *(m)* inferior vestibular nucleus, *(n)* solitary nucleus, *(o)* dorsal motor nucleus X, *(p)* hypoglossal nucleus, *(q)* medial longitudinal fasciculus, *(r)* descending nucleus and tract of trigeminal nerve.

Paramedian medullary syndrome: *(1)* contralateral hemiparesis, *(2)* contralateral hemihypesthesia, *(3)* nystagmus, *(4)* ipsilateral paralysis and atrophy of one half of the tongue.

Lateral medullary (Wallenberg's syndrome): *(5)* ipsilateral hemiataxia, *(6)* Horner's syndrome, *(7)* palatal and vocal cord weakness, *(8)* nystagmus, *(9)* ipsilateral loss of temperature and pain over face and contralateral loss over limbs and trunk.

Circulatory Disorders of the Brainstem

The basal parts of the brain are supplied chiefly by the two vertebral arteries, which join to form the basilar artery. Circulatory disturbances (5–10% of all circulatory disorders) are especially associated with lesions of these arteries and their branches.

BASILAR ARTERY SYNDROME (see also p. 138)

Occlusion of the trunk of the basilar artery—usually by arteriosclerosis with secondary arterial thrombosis—produces the most severe deficits. It leads to softening of the medulla oblongata, pons and midbrain: initially, the patient may retain consciousness, but tetraplegia, and bilateral cranial nerve palsies soon supervene, and the condition is rapidly fatal. *Vertebrobasilar insufficiency* is characterized by transient cranial nerve palsies (double vision), rotatory vertigo or unsteadiness of gait and/or by transient blurring of vision or nausea, which often appears after considerable head movement during housework or daily labor. Sensory disturbances and tetra/hemiparesis may also occur. Occlusions of branches of the basilar artery (or infarcts caused by hemodynamic disturbances) produce unmistakable symptoms, such as *alternating hemiplegia* (clinical types, see p. 125). The predominance of a motor deficit indicates a basal (paramedian) lesion and the predominance of sensory defects points to a lateral infarct. The most common is *Wallenberg's syndrome:* occlusion of the posterior inferior cerebellar artery (or infarction within its territory due to occlusion of the vertebral artery) causes rotatory vertigo, vomiting, hoarseness, nystagmus. It may be accompanied by *Horner's syndrome* (constricted pupil, ptosis, enophthalmos), trigeminal pain and hypesthesia, palatal and deglutition paralysis and ataxia of the extremities. A dissociated centralateral hemiphypesthesia may be present below the neck; also mild motor deficits. The full-blown syndrome is rare, but the prognosis here is better.

Treatment: See cerebral circulatory disturbances.

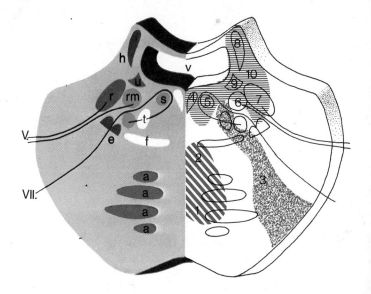

FIG. 54.—Transverse section of the pons. (a) corticospinal tract, (e) lateral lemniscus and lateral spinothalamic tract, (f) medial lemniscus, (h) superior cerebellar peduncle, (m) motor and (r) principal sensory nuclei of trigeminal nerve, (s) abducens nucleus and genu of facial nerve, (t) central tegmental tract, (u) lateral vestibular nucleus, (v) 4th ventricle.

Paramedian pontine syndrome: (1) hemiparesis, (2) hemi-dyssynergia.

Lateral pontine syndrome: (3) hemi-dyssynergia (ipsilateral adiadodyskinesia.

Lateral tegmental pontine syndrome: (4) horizontal gaze paresis, (5) abducens paresis, (6) masticatory paralysis, (7) Horner's syndrome, (8) hemiataxia, (9) vertical nystagmus, (10) intention tremor (according to Hassler).

Name of Syndrome	Ipsilateral Disturbance	Contralateral Disturbance
Medulla Oblongata Syndromes		
Jackson's syndrome	12th (11th, 10th) nerves	Hemiparesis (hemihypesthesia)
Schmidt's syndrome	10th and 11th (12th) nerves	Hemiparesis (hemihypesthesia)
Avellis' syndrome	9th and 10th nerves	Hemiparesis (hemihypesthesia)
Vernet's syndrome	9th, 10th and 11th nerves	Hemiparesis
Céstan-Chenais' syndrome	9th and 10th nerves, ataxia, Horner's syndrome	Hemiparesis (hemihypesthesia)
Babinski-Nageotte's syndrome	Ataxia, Horner's syndrome	Hemiparesis (hemihypesthesia)
Tapia's syndrome	10th and 12th nerves	Hemiparesis (hemihypesthesia)
Wallenberg's syndrome	5th, 9th and 10th nerves, ataxia, Horner's syndrome	Dissociated hemihypesthesia (hemiparesis)
Pontotegmental Syndromes		
Raymond-Céstan's syndrome	6th nerve (gaze paralysis, ataxia)	Hemihypesthesia (hemiparesis)
Gasperini's syndrome	5th–8th nerves (gaze paralysis)	Hemihypesthesia
Foville's syndrome	6th (7th) nerves (gaze paralysis)	Hemiparesis
Millard-Gubler's syndrome	6th and 7th nerves	Hemiparesis
Brissaud's syndrome	Facial hemispasm	Hemiparesis
Parinaud's syndrome	Anterior quadrigeminal bodies	Paralysis of upward gaze
Red Nucleus Syndromes		
Chiray-Foix-Nicolesco syndrome		Hemiparesis, hemichorea, hemiataxia
Benedikt's syndrome	3d nerve	Tremor, hemichorea, ataxia
Weber's syndrome	3d nerve	Hemiparesis
Claude's syndrome	3d nerve	Hemiparesis, hemiataxia, rigidity
Nothnagel's syndrome	3d nerve, hemiataxia	—

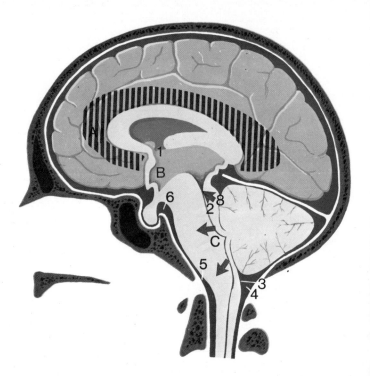

FIG. 55.—Effect of cerebellar spongioblastoma (cerebellar astrocytoma): 4th ventricle and aqueduct are compressed, causing obstruction of the CSF pathways and pressure symptoms. Later, the pons, lower cranial nerves and pyramidal tract are involved (ipsilateral pyramidal signs). The nuclear portion of the vestibular nerve usually is affected early, causing ataxia and nystagmus.

POSTERIOR FOSSA TUMORS (TUMORS OF THE 4TH VENTRICLE)

Etiology: The most common is *cerebellar astrocytoma* (about 30%), occurring especially around the 16th year, and the next most frequent is medulloblastoma (25%), which affects younger children. According to Zülch, the frequency of other infratentorial space-occupying processes is: *angioblastoma* (11%), *ependymoma* (11%), meningioma (5%), arachnoiditis (5%), metastases (2.5%). Rarer lesions are: *choroid plexus papilloma, granuloma* and *capillary hemangioblastoma (von Hippel-Lindau's disease).* The author's personal experience indicates cerebellar metastases are more common, many cases of which are seen in domiciliary consultations.

Clinical: Early clinical features may be occipital headaches and a curious forced posture of the head forward or to one side. Ataxia, asynergy, dysdiadochokinesia and incoordination are comparatively slight; in cerebellar hemisphere lesions, these signs occur ipsilaterally. Gait ataxia may be the only clinical evidence of vermis tumors (medulloblastoma). Compression of the brainstem may lead to a spastic hemi- or tetraplegia. Subsequently, obstruction of the CSF pathways leads to signs of raised intracranial pressure: projectile vomiting without any preliminary choking sensation and especially with sudden movements (e.g., morning rising), *papilledema* and clouded sensorium. CT scanning or echoencephalography reveals a dilated 3d ventricle, and carotid angiography shows a wideswept course of the anterior cerebral artery and dilatation of the lateral ventricles. The skull roentgenograms of children and adolescents may show diastasis of the cranial sutures.

Treatment: Cerebellar astrocytomas are amenable to operative resection; removal of a large part of the cerebellum can be tolerated. Angioblastomas and meningiomas are also operable. Medulloblastomas should be treated by x-irradiation, perhaps combined with attempted surgical excision. Ventricular drainage may be indicated. If no effective treatment is instituted, signs of tonsillar herniation will appear, which progress rapidly to respiratory and circulatory failure.

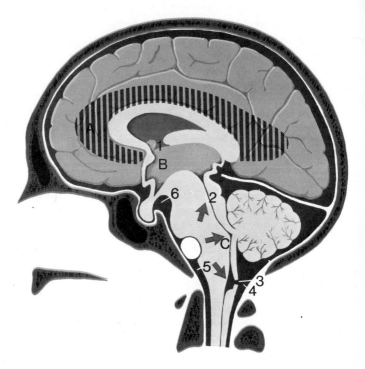

Fig. 56.—Cerebellopontine angle tumors involve early the ipsilateral 5th, 6th, 7th and 8th cranial nerves. A progressive cranial nerve palsy—especially slowly progressive unilateral loss of hearing—should raise this possibility. A clivus meningioma may damage the pyramidal tracts early. Both acoustic neurinomas and meningiomas compress the 4th ventricle and aqueduct, leading to CSF outflow obstruction and raised intracranial pressure.

CEREBELLOPONTINE ANGLE TUMORS

Etiology: The most common (80%) are schwannomas of the vestibular nerve—invariably referred to incorrectly as *acoustic neurinomas*. They may occur in subjects aged 20–60 years and are most frequent in women (2:1). Occasionally, when they are a manifestation of generalized neurofibromatosis (von Recklinghausen's disease), they may be bilateral. A similar clinical picture is produced by *clivus meningiomas* (about 6%), epidermoids (4%), metastases, *chordomas, medulloblastomas, ependymomas,* arteriovenous malformations and granulomatous (adhesive) inflammatory processes.

Clinical: Vertigo is completely absent; however, the otologist may find reduced or absent function of the vestibular nerve. Tinnitus follows and, later, progressive deafness. Only at this stage are the adjacent cranial nerves affected: abducent palsy (double vision on lateral gaze), ipsilateral facial palsy and trigeminal sensory loss (hypesthesias). The corneal reflex is lost. Ipsilateral ataxia follows later (vascular-mediated, or due to pressure on the cerebellus), headache radiating to the occiput and shoulders, ipsilateral (or contralateral) pyramidal disturbances and raised intracranial pressure. Usually *papilledema* and vomiting are present. During the initial stages, the CSF protein level may be normal, but subsequently—it is almost always elevated. In the presence of raised intracranial pressure, lumbar puncture is contraindicated. *Frontal tomography and Stenver's projections* reveal a widened internal auditory canal and bone erosion. Pneumoencephalographic visualization of the cerebellopontine angle and filling of the ventricular system with positive contrast medium outlines the tumor. However, CT or radionuclide scanning, both noninvasive investigative methods, may image it better. Vertebral angiography will exclude an arteriovenous malformation.

Treatment: The only possible treatment is excision of the tumor. The longer the delay and the greater the number of signs of local pressure on adjacent structures the more hazardous the operation. Hearing loss on the side operated on is inevitable.

Review of Extrapyramidal Syndromes

Name of Syndrome	Main Clinical Features	Etiology (Chief Causes)
Parkinson's syndrome	Rigidity, tremor, poverty of movement, bradykinesia, amimia, micrographia, loss of postural reflexes	Epidemic encephalitis: idiopathic, degenerative arteriosclerosis, trauma, etc.
Chorea	Abrupt truncal movements, grimaces	Hereditary, rheumatic fever, pregnancy, etc.
Athetosis	Slow sustained movements of extremeties, postural defects	Brain damage in early life, vascular lesions, metabolic diseases, etc.
(Hemi-)ballismus	Gross flailing movements of one (or more) extremeties	Vascular lesions, tumors, encephalitis, metabolic diseases
Torsion dystonia	Slow rotatory movements around the long axis of the body	Degenerative and hereditary diseases, vascular lesions, tumors, neurosyphilis

Note: Extrapyramidal syndromes initially should be reviewed solely as topographic disorders. Etiologic considerations often require extensive diagnotic investigation and the exclusion of many alternatives in the differential diagnosis.

Parkinson's Syndrome (Paralysis Agitans)

About 11% of the population suffer from this extrapyramidal syndrome of rigidity and poverty of movement.

Etiology: Atrophy of the ganglion cells and neuroglial proliferation, especially of the *substantia nigra*, globus pallidus and corpus striatum, with a reduced *dopamine content* in these structures. The syndrome is inherited as an autosomal dominant disease in about 5–10%, following *encephalitis lethargica* (von Economo) (previously exceeded 60%, now less frequent), as one of the disturbances of cerebral arterial sclerosis (about 20%, now more frequent), after benzol and CO poisoning, cerebral trauma, brain tumors (very rarely), neurosyphilis, etc. Often the cause is never found. A parkinsonian syndrome of moderate severity may follow medication with neuroleptics.

Clinical: The fully developed picture is unmistakable. Typical features are the following: amimia, especially akinesia or hypokinesia, a mask-like expression and seborrheic face, soft staccato speech with repetitive phrases (palilalia), flexed posture (head bent forward), arms flexed, increased tone of both agonistic and antagonistic muscles, rigidity and the cogwheel phenomenon, rhythmic (4–7 seconds) resting tremor of fingers and hands ("pill rolling" or "counting money"), shuffling gait and movements characterized by a tendency to lean forward, backward and sometimes even sideways, coupled with the inability to slow down. The patient's handwriting is small (micrographia) and evidences no tremor. Mental slowing (bradyphrenia) is obvious; affect is flat and labile. Paranoid features, hallucinatory syndromes and psychoses may be present; also an excess of saliva (increased secretion, reduced swallowing) and oculogyric crises, particularly in postencephalitic parkinsonism). Pyramidal tract signs may occur. The parkinsonian crisis consists of extreme poverty of movement, rigidity and fever.

Treatment: The rigidity may be modified by Artane, Akineton, Cogentin, etc., the akinesia by L-dopa. Stereotactic operations on the ventrolateral nucleus of the thalamus reduce the tremor and operations on the globus pallidus diminish the rigidity. Such operations are particularly indicated in cases of unilateral disease and in younger patients (see also p. 134).

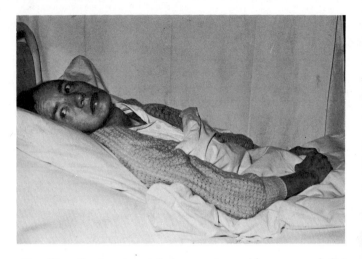

Fig. 57.—Oculogyric crisis in a patient with postencephalitic parkinsonism. This picture, combined with an increased flow of saliva, is found only in the postencephalitic form of the parkinsonism (following epidemic encephalitis or encephalitis lethargica); the latent period separating the initial infection and the oculogyric crisis may be years or even decades. Similar acutely occurring dystonic reactions, especially affecting the mouth, pharynx and neck may be seen after treatment with neuroleptics.

Hyperkinetic Syndromes

CHOREA

Etiology: There are various causes of the underlying lesion of the caudate nucleus (and putamen): *Huntington's chorea* is inherited as an autosomal dominant disease and appears between the ages of 30 and 50 years. *Sydenham's chorea* complicates rheumatic fever in children and young subjects. Similar choreiform hyperkinetic syndromes may accompany pregnancy (and, by analogy, use of ovulation inhibitors) and follow encephalitic illnesses, vascular lesions and (rarely) metastases and primary tumors involving the basal ganglia.

Clinical: Abrupt purposeless involuntary movements of the head and limbs are present during wakefulness and are accentuated by stimulation; they disappear during sleep. Huntington's chorea is a slowly progressive disease and apparent remissions are only temporary, whereas Sydenham's chorea may regress completely within weeks or months; both varieties may present a grotesque clinical picture of constantly changing movements affecting different parts of the body at irregular intervals. Gordon's knee phenomenon is found on testing the knee jerk: with the patient seated with his feet off the floor, relaxation of the limb after contraction is abnormally prolonged. The tongue involvement is noted as clicking sounds during speech. The patient's handwriting is large and flowing. Mental changes accompany Huntington's chorea; later, the patient often is demented. CT and pneumoencephalographic imaging reveals atrophy of the basal ganglia.

Treatment: Neuroleptics and ataractics. Physiotherapy.

ATHETOSIS

Etiology: This clinical picture usually is caused by damage to the globus pallidus (and corpus striatum) early in life, which leaves glial scars that interfere with the transmission of physiologic impulses. *Status marmoratus* often is the end result of perinatal asphyxia. *Status dysmyelinatus* may be a hereditary (autosomal recessive) disease.

Clinical: Continuous, slow, worm-like movements of the legs, forearms and hands with the fingers in fixed positions ("bayonet finger") and "chronic" Babinski signs. See table on page 134.

As a general rule, begin slowly, increase dose carefully until beneficial effect is achieved or another preparation is substituted.

The Brady kinesia responds to L-dopa preparations, Amantidine hydrochloride (Symmetrel).

Significant adverse effects: Dry mouth, disturbance of ocular accommodation and difficulties of micturition and mental confusion are typical of anticholinergics, i.e., Artane, Akineton, Cogentin, Kemadrin and Persidol. Vomiting, nausea, cardiac irregularities, hypotension and dyskinesia may be associated with L-dopa. Edema and livido reticulens may occur following Amantadine.

Treatment of Extrapyramidal Syndromes
CAUSAL: At present, none.
SYMPTOMATIC: Surgical—atereotactic operation in hemiparkin-
           sonian syndromes. Medical.
Parkinson's syndrome: (see Voller, *Aktuelle Neurologie* 1:99 (1974)

Drug	Daily Dosage Range*	Effect on Rigidity	Tremor	Akinesia
Trihexyphenidyl hydrochloride (Artone)	6–15 mg	2+	+	0
Biperiden (Akineton)	2–12 mg	2+	+	(+)
Benztropine (Congentin)	2–6 mg	2+	+++	0
Procyclidine (Kemadrin)	1–20 mg	2+	+	0
Ethopropazine (Persidol)	50–200 mg	0	+++	0
Lerodopa (Larodopa, Dopar)	500–8000 mg	++	+	+++
Lerodopa with carbidopa (Sinemet)	100/10 mg tabs 250/25 mg tabs (3–8 tabs)	+++	+	++++
Amantadine hydrochloride (Symmetrel)	100–200 mg	+	+	++

*(According to: New England Journal of Med: 287:20–24, 1972; & Manual of Neurologic Therapeutics, Boston: Little & Brown, 1978).

HEMIBALLISMUS

Etiology: A lesion of the opposite subthalamic nucleus (corpus Luysii) and less frequently of the corpus striatum and globus pallidus. The underlying cause usually is a vascular insult, rarely a tumor or other lesion.

Clinical: Arrhythmic, violent flailing movements of one side of the body. Those movements affect the proximal joints and they may be sufficiently violent for the patient to lose his balance and injure himself. They are aggravated by excitement and subside during sleep.

Torsion Dystonia (Spasmodic Torticollis)

Etiology: A lesion of the putamen (and globus pallidus), which may be the end result of encephalitis, kernicterus, neonatal asphyxia, an arteriovenous malformation of the basal ganglia, a recessive (or dominant) hereditary disease, "idiopathic" or a manifestation of Kinnier-Wilson's disease (see below).

Clinical: Slow, powerful movements that rotate the patient around the long axis of his body. The muscles of the trunk and proximal extremities are affected most often. In torticollis, the neck muscles contract slowly and rotate the neck by overcoming the opposing force of the antagonist muscles. The disease may begin in early childhood, in youth or in middle age. The prognosis depends on the etiology.

Treatment: Neuroleptics, stereotactic operation.

Hepatolenticular Degeneration (Kinnier-Wilson's disease)

Etiology: An autosomal recessive defect of ceruloplasmin metabolism impairs the transport of copper in the peripheral blood, leading to the deposition of copper in the liver, kidneys, eyes, brain (putamen, globus pallidus), etc., and to excessive excretion of copper in the urine. The serum copper content is reduced (normal: 1.10 mg/liter, range: 0.77–1.85 mg/liter.

Clinical: The disease appears in adolescence (only rarely earlier or later), and the clinical picture is dominated by a cirrhosis of the liver or by signs of extrapyramidal involvement—rigidity, dysarthria, amimia and wing-flapping tremor. These features amount to a choreiform, torsion-dystonic or Parkinsonian syndrome. Mental changes and even dementia are common. Without treatment, the disease is fatal. Copper deposits may be visible in the cornea (Kayser-Fleischer rings).

Treatment: Maintenance treatment with a copper-free diet, calcium sulfide to prevent copper absorption from the gut and D-penicillamine may control the disease or even promote recovery.

135

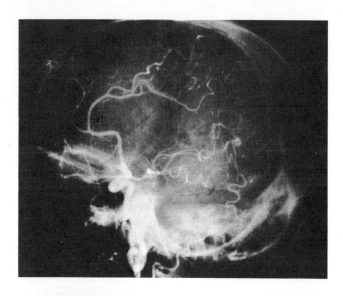

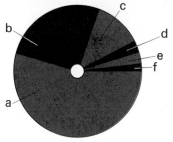

Fig. 58. — *Roentgenogram:* Occlusion of middle cerebral artery. *Diagram:* Incidence of occlusion of cerebral vessels (after Gänshirt): *(a)* Internal carotid artery. *(b)* Middle cerebral artery. *(c)* Posterior cerebral artery. *(d* and *e)* Anterior cerebral artery. *(f)* Basilar artery. Transient ischemic attacks may precede the final event, viz., infarction. Emboli may recur.

Diseases of the Cerebral Circulation

DISTURBANCES OF CEREBRAL PERFUSION (see also p. 123)

Etiology: Most lesions occur as a consequence of arteriosclerosis; only rarely are the causes (circumscribed) endarteritis or panarteritis (sometimes *Horton's giant cell arteritis*). Intimadema or a thrombosis may narrow the lumen severely enough to cause cerebral hypoxia. This leads to cerebral infarction or softening. Embolism is frequent also—systemic emboli especially after myocardial infarction or so-called vitium cordis emboli arising from an ulcerated atheromatous plaque at the carotid bifurcation. The zone of infarction seldom corresponds precisely to the territory of supply of the occluded artery: local perfusion conditions differ greatly; therefore, the clinical picture varies. For example: poor collateral circulation deprives the border zone between two circulatory territories—the "border zone" phenomenon *(Letzten Wiese)*—and "steal" mechanisms may remove oxygenated blood from an area and provoke clinical deficits—the "Robin Hood phenomenon"—leading to a compensatory dilation of vessels within a high-risk territory. Moderate hypoxia (below 50% oxygen supply) may lead to a breakdown of the functional metabolism of the ganglion cells; severe hypoxia (below 15% oxygen available) provokes a total failure of metabolism. Precipitating factors: arterial hypertension and diabetes mellitus. Age of predilection: 50–60 years.

Clinical: Embolism rapidly causes cerebral infarction, especially after strenuous exercise. Arteriosclerosis produces effects more slowly and often at night (hypotension). An immediate flaccid paralysis with pyramidal signs ("apoplexy") is present, later developing into a spastic hemi(mono)plegia(paresis). Individual syndromes of this type may be distinguished, viz.: the *middle cerebral artery syndrome* (50% of cases of "apoplexy"), comprising paralysis and (usually) sensory impairment in the contralateral limbs (the arm more affected than the leg) and the face. Babinski's sign is present. If the dominant hemisphere is affected, aphasia, apraxia, agraphia, alexia and aculculia may occur. In the *anterior cerebral artery syndrome* (5%), the paralysis affects the contralateral lower limb and the patient may exhibit mental changes ("confusion"). In the *posterior cerebral artery syndrome* (about 10%), a contralateral homonymous hemianopia is present, in addition to contralateral sensory changes and if the nondominant hemisphere is

137

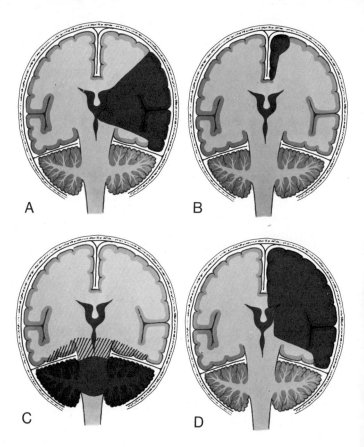

Fig. 59.—Zones of infarction following complete occlusion of middle cerebral artery **(A)**, anterior cerebral artery **(B)**, basilar artery **(C)** and internal carotid artery **(D)**. The clinical deficits seldom are so extensive, since the boundary zones of each territory are irrigated by the vessels supplying the adjacent territory. This applies also to occlusions of branches of the main trunks. A collateral blood supply may also be delivered via leptomeningeal anastamoses, the circle at Willis and, if present via persisting primitive arteries. In anterior cerebral artery occlusion (involvement of paracentral lobule syndromes), sphincteric impairment.

138

affected, unilateral neglect, dressing apraxia, spatial disorientation and constructive apraxia are seen. In the *internal carotid artery syndrome* (most commonly changes in the arterial wall occur at the carotid bifurcation), clinical signs and symptoms of involvement of all three vascular territories are combined; hemianopia is less frequent, perfusion of the occipital territory being maintained by the vertebrobasilar system. Anomalies of the circle of Willis and other factors greatly modify the clinical picture. The occurrence of severe cerebral edema—especially in young subjects—may cause a midbrain syndrome and lead rapidly to death. Increasing clouding of consciousness is a warning sign. As a rule, the ganglion cells recover after the edema has subsided due to an increased blood supply via collateral vessels, normalization of the focal metabolic patterns and functional adaptation to the new situation. A spastic hemiplegia (Wernicke-Mann) is not uncommon—circumduction of the contralateral lower extremity, flexed arms and contracted fingers. Symptoms subside as a rule, in 4–12 weeks, when only mild residual signs remain (less movement on one side, facial asymmetry, etc.).

Diagnosis: Cerebral hemorrhage (prognosis worse; more rapid progression of signs of a space-occupying lesion, often blood-stained CSF, less definite localization with respect to vascular territory) and hemorrhage into tumors (glioblastoma) should be considered. If in doubt, the following investigations may be helpful: EEG (only minor changes in vascular occlusion), CT scanning (low-density area, which may be enhanced with a contrast medium), carotid angiography (site of occlusion directly visible; some inherent risks) or cerebral scintigraphy (positive also in tumors). The extent of cerebral softening, although often quite sizable, often is difficult to determine. The course of the disease is particularly important. Mental symptoms are common.

Treatment: Improving cardiac output (digitalis), countering edema (hyperosmolar solutions), prolonged physiotherapy and treatment of risk factors (hypertension). In individual cases of embolism, anticoagulants may prevent recurrent emboli.

Try substances acting on cerebral metabolism (anthinol niacinate = Complamin, Stutgeron, etc.). Transient ischemic attacks in the carotid territory (focal neurologic deficity lasting less than 12 hours) due to local stenosis or an ulcerated plaque at the carotid befurcation are amenable to surgery (carotid endarterectomy).

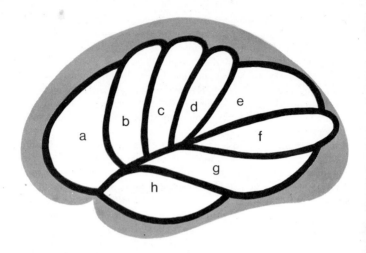

Fig. 60.—Diagrammatic representation of the artial supply of the middle cerebral artery and its branches.

a = orbitofrontal artery
b = prerolandic artery
c = rolandic artery
d = anterior parietal artery
e = posterior parietal artery
f = angular artery
g = posterior temporal artery
h = anterior temporal artery

Syndromes of Cerebral Artery Occlusions

Occluded Artery	Signs
Internal carotid artery	Contralateral hemiplegia, hemi-sensory deficit, homonymous hemianopia, *aphasia, apraxia
Anterior cerebral artery	Contralateral lower limb paresis, loss of sphincter control, lack of initiative and spontaneity.
Middle cerebral artery	Contralateral hemiparesis (involving chiefly face and upper limbs), hemi-sensory deficit, homonymous hemi-anopia, *aphasia, apraxia, and agraphia, anosognosia.
Posterior cerebral artery	Contralateral homonymous hemianopia, occasional object agnosia, alexia without agraphia.
Anterior choroidal artery	Hemiplegia, hemianesthesia, and hemi-anopia.
Prerolandic artery	Focal paresis, non-fluent or (Broca's) motor aphasia.
Anterior temporal artery	Fluent (Wernicke's) aphasia
Anterior parietal artery	Contralateral hemi-sensory deficit, astereognosis.
Angular artery	*Agraphia, acalculia, finger agnosia, right-left disorientation, alexia, apraxia; bodily agnosia, hemi-sensory deficits.

COMMENT

The complete syndromes as outlined are only rarely seen. In practice more often the clinical picture is incomplete, and difficult to localize due to several infarcts (?) or watershed infarcts (?), or alterations of the functional deficits by adaptation of new neuronal pathways (neuroplasticity).

---

*The neuropsychologic deficit attributed solely to the dominant hemisphere are listed.

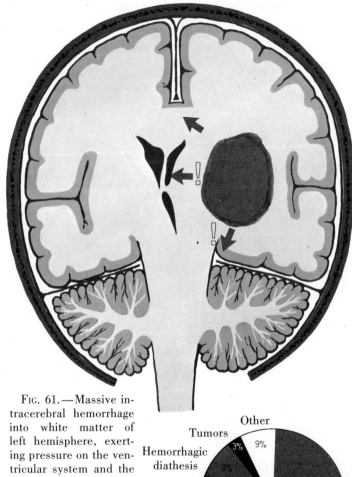

Fig. 61.—Massive intracerebral hemorrhage into white matter of left hemisphere, exerting pressure on the ventricular system and the tentorial notch. Causes of intracerebral hemorrhage are given (%) in the diagram.

Other
Tumors
9%
3%
Hemorrhagic diathesis
8%
Aneurysms
20%
50%
Hypertension

CEREBRAL HEMORRHAGE (Intracerebral Hematoma)

Etiology: Arteriosclerosis usually is the cause in elderly people. In 60–80% of these patients, preexisting arterial hypertension is present, and the remainder may show evidence of generalized arteriosclerosis (early cerebral infarction, myocardial infarction, intermittant claudication). In each case of intracranial hemorrhage in a young subject, *aneurysm* (it is not always demonstrable by angiography) or *arteriovenous malformation* must be excluded. In older subjects, glioblastoma multiforme is a not infrequent cause of cerebral hemorrhage. *Anticoagulant medications* or hematologic diseases (thrombopenia, generalized purpura, etc.) may be a significant factor.

Clinical: Usually after strenuous physical exertion—sometimes only a few days later—a hemiparesis develops over the course of hours, which progresses to hemiplegia, confusion and signs of raised intracranial pressure. Papilledema appears within 2–3 days. The patient may turn his head or eyes to the side of the lesion and exhibit release phenomena (grasp reflex). If bleeding continues, a midbrain syndrome (arrows, Fig. 61) develops, leading to a decerebrate state and death. The CSF need not be bloodstained, even if the hematoma ruptures into the ventricular system—usually a fatal event (early obstruction of CSF pathway). The EEG shows focal delta waves, usually also generalized changes. Echoencephalography reveals a significant midline displacement, and carotid angiography shows the mass to be avascular. The extent of the hematoma and its mass effect on the ventricular system are best shown by CT scanning, since coagulated blood is significantly more dense than normal brain tissue. Arterial hypertension may result from the hemorrhage. Later, the raised intracranial pressure may lead to gastrointestinal hemorrhage (Cushing's ulcer), aspiration pneumonia or circulatory and respiratory paralysis with cerebral death.

Treatment: No treatment can influence the hemorrhage—or stop it. Careful attention to preventing complications and controlling cerebral edema. Operative evacuation should be considered in young subjects and others, if the site is favorable.

Arteriovenous Malformation. An important cause of spontaneous intracerebral hemorrhage is arteriovenous malformation (AVMs). AVMs may be asymptomatic for years or be associated with vascular headaches (migraine). Later, however, episodes of

143

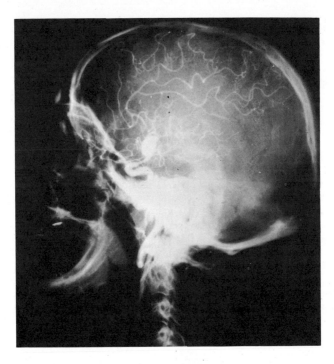

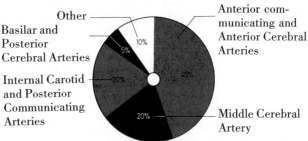

Fig. 62.—*Roentgenogram:* left carotid angiogram showing large saccular aneurysm of the anterior communicating artery, the cause of a subarachnoid hemorrhage. *Diagram:* Frequency of occurrence of aneurysms on various cerebral arteries (according to Schiefer in Gänshirt).

acute intraparenchymal cerebral hemorrhage or progressive focal neurologic deficits may occur. Cerebral angiography reveals the site and the extent of the vascular malformation. Complete surgical extirpation or partial obliteration by embolization of feeding arteries are therapeutic approaches.

Subarachnoid Hemorrhage (Cerebral Aneurysms)

Etiology: Saccular intracranial aneurysms are a chance finding in about 1% of all autopsies—significantly even more common are muscular (tunica media) defects, which form the basis of most aneurysms. The most common site is the anterior communicating artery, then the bifurcation of the internal carotid and the proximal portions of the middle and posterior cerebral arteries, i.e., the posterior communicating artery. Arterial hypertension, strenuous exercise, etc., are likely to transform the media defect to an aneurysm, causing it to rupture into the subarachnoid space and/or plow a track through the adjacent brain substance; soon, the blood diffuses throughout the subarachnoid space. A rarer cause of aneurysm is arteriosclerosis; syphilis is almost never a cause. Common in young persons.

Clinical: Usually after exertion, the patient experiences a severe local headache, which spreads over the entire vertex and down the spine. Vagal stimulation commonly leads to vomiting, and unconsciousness follows an extensive hemorrhage. The admixture of blood and CSF in the subarachnoid space leads to moderate fever, neck stiffness and nerve root irritation. The clinical picture mimics meningitis. Subhyloid retinal hemorrhages are present. After some weeks, the temperature falls, the frankly blood-stained CSF becomes xanthochromic and then clear; the CSF picture returns to normal after phagocytosis of red cells and an admixture of hemosiderin phagocytes (with slight pleocytosis). High risk of recurrence. The first hemorrhage may be, the second often is, and the third always is fatal.

Treatment: Strict bed rest with sedation is essential following the attack, reduction of elevated blood pressure and prevention of other external stimuli. All strenuous activities must be minimized (attention to defecation). When the patient's general condition permits, four-vessel cerebral arteriography (carotid and vertebral) to demonstrate the aneurysm or other cause of hemorrhage must be undertaken. Thereafter, immediate operation! Aneurysms may be multiple.

145

Causes of Purulent Meningitis: Bacteria
(Average values from numerous series in the literature)

Meningococci   20–50%
Pneumococci   15–35%
Hemophilus influenzae   2–20%
Streptococci   2–10%
Staphylococci   1–9%
Escherichia coli   1%
Very Rare:

Listeria monocytogenes	*Pseudomomas aeruginosa*
Salmonella cholerae suis	*Proteus vulgaris*
Aerobacter aerogenes	*Neisseria gonorrhoeae*
Neisseria catarrhalis	*Brucella melitensis, abortis, suis*
Klebsiella pneumoniae	*Corynebacterium diphtheriae*

Causes of Lymphocytic Meningitis

Viruses:	Mumps (epidemic parotitis)	Coxsackie group
	Poliomyelitis	Herpes zoster
	St. Louis encephalitis	Encephalitis japonica
	Rabies	Herpes simplex
	Louping ill meningitis	Encephalitis epidemica
	Echovirus group	Lymphocytic choriomeningitis
	Central European encephalitis	Infectious mononucleosis, etc.
	Ornithosis (psittacosis)	
	Influenza	
Bacteria:	Tuberculosis	*Bacterium tularense*
	Leptospirosis	Brucelloses
	Treponema pallidum	Salmonelloses
Protozoa:	Toxoplasmosis	*Plasmodium malariae*
	Trypanosoma gambiense	*Naegleria*, etc.
Fungi:	Actinomycosis	Cryptococcosis (torulosis)
	Histoplasmosis	Moniliasis, etc.
Parasites:	Echinococcosis	Schistosomiasis
	Trichinosis	Cysticercosis
	Paragonimiasis	

Inflammatory Diseases of the Brain

MENINGITIDES (MENINGOENCEPHALITIDES)

Etiology: Meningitis has many causes. Apart from numerous bacteria, treponemes, viruses, fungi, protozoa and parasites, it may be produced by chemical substances; e.g., cholesteatoma rupturing into the CSF. Also collagenoses and etiologically ill defined processes such as *sarcoidosis*, the *Melkersson-Rosenthal syndrome* and Behçet's disease may be accompanied by meningitis. The infective agent may reach the CSF compartment via the blood stream (hematogenous) or through contiguous tissues—*sinogenic* and *otogenic* meningitis are important entities. Recent trauma (compound craniocerebral injuries, but also simple fractures of the skull base) allow CSF to escape via the paranasal sinuses and ears (confirm CSF fistula, viz., rhinorrhea or otorrhea by the glucose test: the escaping fluid contains glucose) and microorganisms enter the leptomeningeal spaces. In old injuries, microorganisms may remain dormant for a long time and become active if the patient's body resistance falls: meningitis and especially brain abscess result.

Meningococci are the most common cause of bacterial meningitis (40% in children, 20% in adults), pneumococci (20% in children, 30% in adults), *H. influenzae* (10%), streptococci (about 8%) and staphylococci (about 5%). Less frequent: *Salmonella, Listeria monocytogenes, Pseudomonas aeruginosa* (after spinal anesthesia), *Neisseria, Clostridium, Escherichia coli* and *Proteus mirabilis.* The *leptospira* may also cause meningitis, including *Treponema pallidum* (see Neurosyphilis, p. 153) and mycobacteria.

Suspicion of a virus infection should prompt consideration of the following: *lymphocytic choriomeningitis* (transmitted by mice), *Central European encephalitis* (transmitted by tick bite), *coxsackie viruses, echoviruses, herpes zoster, herpes simplex* (dangerous encephalitides), *mumps, measles, German measles* and *infectious mononucleosis.*

Amebic meningoencephalitis caused by *Naegleria* may be fatal. *Toxoplasmosis* should be considered. Mycoses usually are a terminal event, in the presence of reduced body resistance and previous antibiotic treatment. Very rarely, *cryptococci* and other fungi may be a primary cause of meningitis (encephalitis). Parasites are rare causes in temperate climates but common in the tropics (eosinophilic meningitis).

147

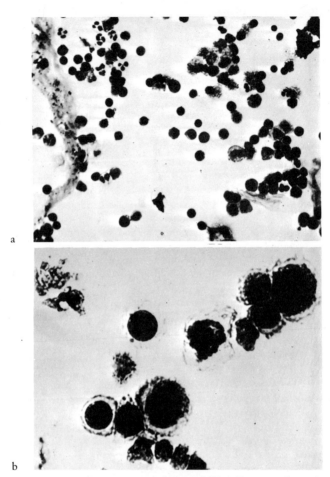

Fig. 63.—Millipore preparation of CSF cells in resolving bacterial meningitis. **(a)** A few polymorphonuclear leukocytes are visible, surrounded by many monocytes and some lymphocytes. Later, the polys disappear completely and the monocytes and lymphocytes slowly diminish. **(b)** Cell picture in carcinomatous meningitis: apart from monocytes, large tumor cells are visible, which possess giant round nuclei, some in mitosis.

148

Clinical: The introduction of microorganisms into the CSF (and the resulting release of reactive substances) leads to prompt dissemination in the leptomeningeal spaces and immune reactions *(pleocytosis and raised protein,* especially globulin fraction). Raised CSF pressure causes *severe headache.* To seek relief, the patient throws his head back *(opisthotonos, neck stiffness)* and draws up his legs. All body movements are painful, all sensory stimuli are unpleasant. Soon, the temperature begins to rise and a very *high fever* ensues. Metabolic derangement of the cerebral cortex (toxic effects, spread of the infection across the blood-brain barrier and by continuity) leads to mental clouding and later to loss of consciousness (coma). The earlier the mental symptoms occur the longer they last and the worse the prognosis. In the bacterial meningitides, a purulent membrane forms over the cerebral hemispheres and at the base of the skull. The blood picture and ESR reflect an acute infective process. The *CSF* is cloudy or purulent. Polymorphonuclear cells are prominent in bacterial infections and in all acute stages of the disease. Viral meningitides (and some other varieties) show lymphatic pleocytosis as high as 2000 cells (bacterial meningitis: up to 60,000). The protein content is greatly increased. Glucose content is depressed in bacterial and fungal conditions. Causal organisms may be cultured from specimens removed before the start of treatment. Unless exceptional circumstances exist, treatment should follow identification of the causal microorganism. Drug sensitivities should be determined also, if at all possible. Finally, the site of entry should be identified and repaired (closure of CSF fistula, drainage of paranasal sinuses).

Prognosis: Meningococcal meningitis responds best to treatment (cure rate over 90%), pneumococcal meningitis less well (mortality about 40%). The prognosis depends largely on the speed with which the initial diagnosis is reached and treatment is started and also on the adequacy of dosage and the length of therapeutic drug treatment. Each hour is valuable.

Guidelines for Treatment of Purulent Meningitides

1. Initiate treatment immediately, once diagnosis is confirmed. Any delay worsens the prognosis. *Spinal tap is necessary to obtain CSF for identifying the causal organism.*

Adults: Penicillin 20–40 million U a day, or ampicillin 12–14 gm a day.

Children: Ampicillin 300–400 mg/kg/day and chloramphenicol 50–100 mg/kg/day.

No later than the 3rd day, the temperature should have fallen to normal; if there is no fall, alter the antibiotic.

2. Following *identification of the causal organism and the determination of the drug sensitivities*, specific therapy should be started immediately:

Meningococci: Additional penicillin or sulfonamide 4–6 gm or chloramphenicol 3 gm a day. Children: 60 mg/kg.

Pneumococci: Penicillin or chloramphenicol 3–4 gm. Children: 70 mg/kg.

H. influenzae: Chloramphenicol 3 gm a day. Children: 60 mg/kg or Ampicillin 12–14 gm/day. Children: 300–400 mg/kg/day.

Streptococci: see Pneumococci.

Staphylococci: Methicillin, oxacillin 8–10 gm a day. Children: 2–4 gm a day. Chloramphenicol 3–4 gm a day. Children: 70 mg/kg.

E. coli: Ampicillin 6–8 a day. Children: 70 mg/kg. Streptomycin 2 gm a day. Children: 50 mg/kg. Chloramphenicol 3–4 gm a day. Children: 70 mg/kg.

Listeria monocytogenes: Ampicillin 6 gm a day. Children: 70 mg/kg or Tetracycline 2 gm a day. Children: 40 mg/kg.

Pseudomonas aeruginosa: Carbenicillin 24–36 gm/day. Children: 400–600 mg/kg/day and Gentamicin 5 mg/kg/day.

Proteus vulgaris: Sulfonamide, streptomycin.

Protozoa: Seek advise from tropical medicine specialist.

Fungi: Cryptococci—amphotericin B 1 mg/kg and 5-fluorocytosine (5-FC) 150 mg kg/day.

Parasites: Seek advise from tropical medicine specialist.

Remarks: In no case should nonspecific treatment be neglected.

> *Cardiac and circulatory support* (? digitalis)
> Adequate *fluid intake* (2–3 liters by infusion)
> Regulate electrolyte balance
> Consider *corticosteroids*

Any efficacious antibiotic may have life-threatening side effects. Dose varies according to individual circumstances.

Treatment: As soon as lumbar puncture reveals the presence of a meningitis in the CSF, large doses of intravenous penicillin (10–40 million units a day) should be administered. If the temperature fails to fall significantly within 2 days or if the nature of the causal organism (and its drug resistances) becomes known, another antibiotic should be substituted. Treatment should continue for 8–14 days following the return of a normal temperature and until all CSF parameters have returned to normal (cell count below 100). If fever and pleocytosis persist despite the administration of several antibiotics, the presence of a fungal infection should be suspected.

Additional Treatment: Cooperation with a good laboratory service is important, including familiarity with the requirements for virologic, mycologic and parasitic investigation. In most countries, infective meningitides, if transmissible, are reportable diseases.

Complications: Localized empyema formation and subsequent CSF pathway obstruction, cranial nerve deficits, thromboangitides with small cerebral infarcts and seizures—the clinical picture varies greatly. Other organs may be involved (pericarditis, pleurisy, peritonitis). Meningococcal meningitis may upset adrenal function, provoking a critical hypotensive state *(Marchand-Waterhouse syndrome)*. Symptomatic psychoses may occur.

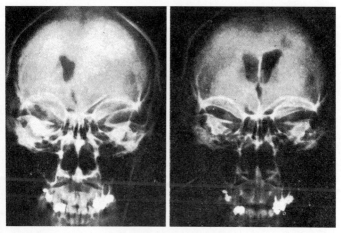

FIG. 64.—Left hemisphere space-occupying lesion **(left)** which regressed completely **(right)** after 20 days of treatment with penicillin and iodides. Syphilitic pseudotumor.

151

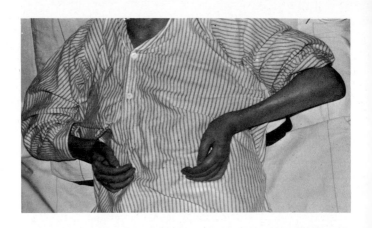

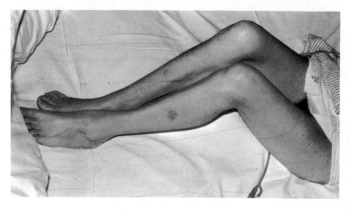

Fig. 65.—Flaccid paralysis and considerable atrophy of muscles of both arms, marked spastic paralysis of the legs and dissociated sensory loss in a patient with leutic anterior spinal artery syndrome involving the C8–T6 segments of the spinal cord. Spastic stage of disease. Bilateral Babinski signs. Contracture of leg muscles.

Neurosyphilis (see also pp. 116 and 117)

The causal organism of syphilis (lues), *Treponema pallidum*, reaches the nervous system during the second stage of the disease. The clinical picture of *early syphilitic meningitis* is characterized by slight neck stiffness, low-grade fever and pleocytosis (lymphocytic predominance). Without treatment, a chronic inflammatory process, *syphilitic meningoencephalitis*, may develop; it extends from the blood vessels *(Heubner's syphilitic endarteritis)* and gives rise to the typical granulomatous lesion of the disease *(gumma)*. Transient pareses accompanying smaller infarcts, as well as various other clinical signs, may complicate the picture; rarely, syphilitic infection may mimic an intracranial tumor. CSF examination is conclusive (infection); also the Wassermann and associated reactions.

Tabes dorsalis occurs 3–20 years after the onset of infection. According to Scheid, the most common early symptoms of tabes are sudden and severe lancinating pains (35%), ataxia due to posterior column atrophy (27%), visual disturbances, including optic atrophy (11%), which may lead to blindness, lower limb weakness (4%), vertigo (2%), bladder disturbances (1.3%) and hypersensitivity to cold (0.6%). The pupils react poorly (or not at all) to light, but normally to convergence (Argyll Robertson pupil). Truncal hyperpathia and segmental (root) hypesthesia are found: the deep tendon reflexes are reduced or absent and there is gross sensory ataxia and defective locomotor control, which increases when visual cues are absent in darkness. Joint deformities frequently develop. Sometimes spontaneous fractures and painless perforating skin ulcers *(mal perforant)* are seen. In 70% of patients, serologic test for syphilis (UDRL) is positive in the blood and also in the CSF, which shows a mild lymphocytic pleocytosis and raised protein (globulin) level.

Guidelines for Treatment of Neurosyphilis

1. *Adequate diagnostic confirmation* by serologic test for syphilis (or other test) in blood and CSF; also treponemal test (TTA-abs).
   In doubtful cases, repeat investigations. Decide whether nonspecific positive reactions are significant.
2. *Penicillin* 1 million units IM daily for 15 days followed by a 14-day rest period. Then 2–4 further courses, the last one after a 3-month rest. Evaluate progress by CSF examinations, the first 4 weeks after the start of treatment and the last 1–2 years after the end of treatment.
   Cases of penicillin sensitivity (rare): tetracycline 1 gm daily for 14 days.

Guidelines for Treatment of Tuberculosis

1. Confirm the diagnosis by direct observation of the causal organism in a CSF smear (Ziehl-Neelsen stain), culture (egg medium) and/or animal inoculation (guinea pigs). Other microorganisms invariably must be considered; also *sarcoidosis* and collagenoses.
2. Treatment with triple-drug combination. Start with
   streptomycin 1.5–2 gm a day. Children: 30–40 mg/kg up to 30–40 gm.
   INH 10–15 mg/kg a day up to 40–50 gm.
   PAS 20–24 gm a day by infusion for 30 days, then 8–12 gm by mouth in 2–3 hours.
Later, these preparations must be replaced by
   rifampin 5–10 mg/kg by mouth up to 6 months, or
   ethambutol 15–25 mg/kg by mouth up to 3 months, or
   ethionamide 0.75–1 gm a day up to 2 months, or
   cycloserine 3–4 × 250 mg a day up to 3 months, etc.
Intravenous treatment should be varied, due to the development of resistance to various drugs. *All efficacious antibiotics may produce severe side-effects. Observe contraindications*, individual dose schedules.

An important symptom for which the patient invariably seeks medical help is the "tabetic crisis," a very painful and frightening attack in which shooting pains may involve the abdomen (gastric crisis), throat, parotid, kidneys, ureter, bladder or urethra.

Treatment: At least 3 consecutive courses of treatment with penicillin 1 million units a day for 15 days. Complete normalization of the CSF should be the therapeutic goal. Keep the patient under observation for years.

GENERAL PARESIS (DEMENTIA PARALYTICA)

This progressive cerebral disorder develops 8–20 years after the initial infection. It is characterized by various mental deficits: the patient becomes less observant, his effort and drive are blunted, his memory becomes poor and his personality changes. A well-marked psychotic state may develop, with the patient exhibiting paranoid, depressive or (rarely) manic features. The underlying lesion is a smoldering infective process near the cerebral cortex, which causes thickening of the pia and arachnoid membranes, degeneration of ganglion cells, glial proliferation and disorganization of the normal lamination of the cerebral cortex. An increase in the iron content of glial cells and a mesenchymal phagocytosis are demonstrable by special staining methods. In a focal variety, *Lissauer's paralysis,* the disease is confined to individual parts of the brain (temporal lobe, parietal lobe).

Typical neurologic signs may be minimal or absent: abnormal pupil, including *Argyll Robertson's sign,* transient weaknesses caused by small-vessel occlusions, brisk reflexes and pyramidal signs, jacksonian attacks, bladder disturbances, etc. Dysarthria and anarthria are frequent. The patient exhibits a remarkably vacant facial expression, due to abnormal flaccidity of the facial muscles, and a perioral "tremor" often is present when the patient speaks. The CSF shows a pleocytosis, increased globulin and marked leftward deviation of the colloidal gold curve. Serologic test for syphilis (VDRL) is positive.

Treatment: Courses of high-dose penicillin, perhaps combined with fever therapy. In any neurologic disease of questionable etiology, consider neurosyphilis.

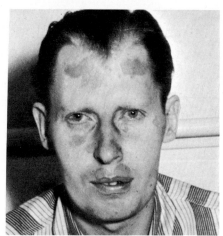

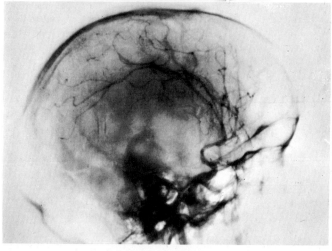

Fig. 60.—Neurosarcoidosis commencing as a florid cutaneous disease (Heerfort's syndrome, viz., fever, uveitis, parotitis, facial palsy) and developing via a lymphocytic meningitis to cerebral atrophy and tetraspasticity. Mantoux test negative. Carotid angiogram reveals a temporal lobe mass, which proved to be a sarcoid granuloma.

Tuberculosis of the Nervous System

Tuberculous meningitis is a not uncommon manifestation of generalized spread of the disease: it occurs in 75% of cases of miliary tuberculosis. Nonspecific signs such as neck stiffness, fever, headache and confusion are accompanied by cranial nerve palsies (double vision)—tuberculous meningitis attacks the base of the brain. The CSF shows a pleocytosis (up to 1000 cells), a high protein content (up to 300 mg/100ml), spontaneous clotting on standing, xanthochromia and—following staining with Ziehl-Neelsen's reagent and as a reward for prolonged searching—mycobacteria. The inevitably poor prognosis of previous years has been transformed by the introduction of streptomycin (*warning:* toxic vestibular nerve damage with 30 gm!), INH (*warning:* polyneuritis—therefore, always combine with vitamin B_6!), PAS (24 gm daily by infusion) and other antitubercular drugs. Treatment is necessary for many months. Complications due to adhesions (CSF pathway obstruction) and spread to cerebral blood vessels—hydrocephalus is a common late effect (see p. 121). *Tuberculomas* are rare, occurring in the so-called tertiary stage of the disease (organ tuberculosis) and seen on biopsy as an intracranial space-occupying mass (raised intracranial pressure).

Sarcoidosis and Other Granulomatous Inflammations

Sarcoidosis of the nervous system is one of the most common of the numerous meningitides which are characterized by the following: no demonstrable causal organism, chronic clinical course, intracranial granulomata deforming the CSF pathway and a variable clinical picture—*facial palsy*, pyramidal signs, *seizures*, hypothalamic signs (diabetes insipidus), *papilledema*, ataxia, mental changes and polyneuritis multiplex. A pleocytosis, sarcoid deposits in other organs (skin, lymph nodes, eyes, etc.) and a positive *Kveim test* confirm the diagnosis and indicate treatment with corticosteroids. Obstruction of the CSF pathway necessitates surgical intervention. Focal involvement of the nervous system—and similarly protean signs and symptoms—also accompany Behçet's disease, systemic lupus erythematosus, periarteritis nodosa, etc.

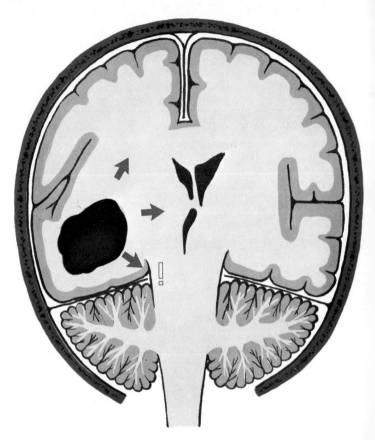

Fig. 67.—Abscesses filled with purulent yellow or greenish yellow material usually develop in the temporal lobe, less often in the cerebellum or brain stem. Initially multilocular, they later develop a connective tissue capsule and assume a spherical shape. Because of their size and the surrounding edema, they mimic brain tumors in exerting a mass effect on the ventricular system and brain stem. Antibiotic instillation into the abscess cavity following surgical drainage!

Encephalitides

Etiology: Many types of meningitis also involve the brain; thus, one speaks of meningoencephalitis in the case of most viral infections of the nervous system. Similarly, the encephalitides, which affect chiefly the brain substance, often involve the meninges; the mildest manifestation is a pleocytosis. The following conditions merit special attention: hemorrhagic *herpes encephalitis*, which starts abruptly and leads to focal brain necrosis (temporal lobe) and death; encephalitis lethargica (von Economo's disease) with an inverted sleep rhythm, external ocular palsies and a secondary *vaccination encephalitis* (incidence 1:100,000). Other encephalitic diseases include *sleeping sickness (Trypanosoma gambiense)* and rabies (hydrophobia, agitation, later external ocular and bulbar palsies and confusion). More common in Western Europe is *Central European encephalitis* (and associated diseases in North America, Japan, etc. transmitted by arthropods). It may not always be possible to identify the causal organism, despite the obvious presence of an infection.

Clinical: The most common features are variation in body temperatures, headache, vomiting, joint pains, photophobia, pyramidal tract signs, cranial nerve palsies and mental disturbances. Seizures and hyperkinetic movements may occur also. The CSF has an increased protein content and cell count (about 1000/mm³ cells). Electroencephalography reveals a generalized dysrhythmia. Signs of raised intracranial pressure, including papilledema, may occur.

Treatment: Symptomatic, and measures to combat the causal agent (see meningitides). Adenine arabinoside (Ara A) for herpes encephalitis.

BACTERIAL ENCEPHALITIS, CEREBRAL ABSCESS

Bacterial cerebritis—often accompanying meningitis—usually represents the intermediate stage in the formation of a brain abscess. The responsible pathogens are staphylococci, streptococci or pneumococci. The clinical features mimic a brain tumor, and include hemiparesis, raised intracranial pressure and seizures. The blood picture and erythrocyte sedimentation rate and sometimes the cellular content of the CSF point to an inflammatory lesion.

Treatment: Operation. Antibiotics (penicillin and chloramphenicol).

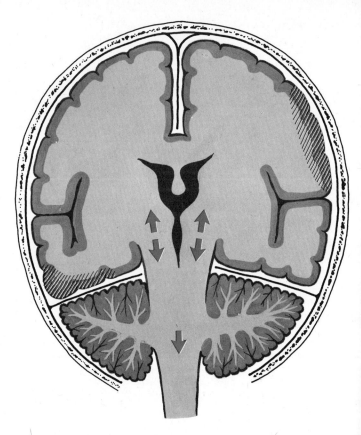

Fig. 68.—Closed craniocerebral trauma is very common. As illustrated in this diagram, the damage may involve the contralateral cortex as well as the brain substance immediately beneath the point of impact. Initially, a small subarachnoid hemorrhage occurs, then a tent-shaped area of cerebral softening, finally fluid-filled cysts with brownish red discoloration of the overlying surface. Sites of predilection: areas in which the subarachnoid space is deficient. Parenchymal damage is favored by rotation or herniation effects accompanying acceleration or deceleration trauma.

Craniocerebral Trauma

Etiology: Annually, about 300,000 head injuries occur in Germany, including 16,000 fatal cases of craniocerebral trauma. The majority are caused by automobile accidents; others are due to sports, work or household injury. Open head injuries may be complicated by further hemorrhage or infection. Closed injuries are more common, and they are classified clinically as: (1) *Commotio cerebri (cerebral concussion)*, which, although causing no histologically detectable brain damage, results in a loss of consciousness lasting up to 2 hours, an autonomic reaction (vomiting, tachycardia, etc.) and *retrograde amnesia*, i.e., the patient is unaware of events that took place during the minutes or hours immediately before the accident. Physical findings are minimal.

Treatment: Consists of bedrest for several days (or weeks). Drug therapy is directed at autonomic stabilization and the symptomatic relief from headache. A quiet atmosphere and cold compresses on the forehead are advisable. Full recovery within 4 (–12) weeks. (2) *Contusio cerebri* (cerebral contusion). Severe head injuries cause focal cortical contusions beneath the site of impact and similar lesions in the opposite cortex (contrecoup). They produce paresis but rarely sensory or visual aphasia. Unconsciousness is present only with concomitant concussion. In *brain stem contusion*, which may threaten life, microhemorrhages and edema lead to unconsciousness lasting hours (days or weeks), severe autonomic disturbances (pyrexia, tachycardia, central respiratory distress, hypotensive crises, etc.) and, subsequently, significant mental changes (contusional psychosis and disorientation, memory disturbance and abnormal affect: the usual picture is one of blunting of affect and lack of spontaneity without disturbances of consciousness). The CSF often is slightly blood-stained. The electroencephalogram may show focal or generalized abnormalities.

Cranial nerve palsies (olfactory, ocular, trochlear, abducent, facial) may be present. Generalized epileptiform seizures ("early traumatic epilepsy") may supervene. Progressive *cerebral edema* (2d–5th day) aggravates the situation. A space-occupying intracerebral mass effect develops if the edema is severe, leading to coma and a *midbrain syndrome*. Complete respiratory depression, circulatory failure and pressure-induced gastric ulcers (Cushing) may end in death. Fluid and electrolyte balance is impaired. Decerebrate posturing (arms flexed or extended, legs extended) with a

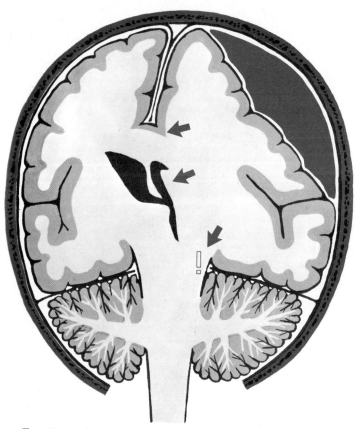

Fig. 69.—A large subdural hematoma accumulates in the course of days or weeks (even months) after craniocerebral trauma, which may be slight. Compression of one or both cerebral hemispheres produces headache and mental symptoms and eventually unconsciousness due to midbrain compression. Carotid angiography reveals displacement of the control vessels from the inner table of the skull. Patients on anticoagulants are at high risk. Immediate surgical evacuation!

stepwise increase in severity is common. Disturbances of sensory function are present and stimulation leads only to extensor spasms. The muscles are spastic and pyramidal signs (Babinski) are present. Improvement is heralded by the appearance of primitive reflexes (lip smacking, rhythmic chewing movements, withdrawal from painful stimuli, snouting). An *apallic syndrome* may develop and the patient becomes an akinetic mute, lying silent and motionless in bed, with eyes open, arms flexed and legs extended, apparently awake, yet not reacting to stimuli ("parasomniac conscious state"). The complications of this state are footdrop, muscle contractures (myositis ossificans) and bedsores. Some improvement may occur but there usually is residual personality change, intellectual poverty (dementia) and hemi- or tetraspasticity. The symptoms and signs of a simple contusion may regress completely within months without residual evidence of a gross deficit. Late (and rare) sequelae include seizures ("post-traumatic epilepsy"), which may appear more than 2 years after injury. EEG follow-up advisable.

Diagnosis: CT scanning, carotid arteriography or echoencephalography to exclude a surgically treatable mass (epi- or subdural or intracerebral hematoma). A purulent meningitis should prompt a search for a (hidden) CSF fistula.

Treatment: 14 days of symptomatic treatment—control of edema, attention to circulation, respiration, fluid and electrolyte balance. Intravenous or tube feeding. Quiet surroundings, physiotherapy. Intensive nursing care. Later, anticonvulsants. Treatment of hyperthermia (icepacks), hypothermia and peripheral circulatory stimulation with Complamin. Assisted respiration may be necessary. Dexamethasone is indicated to reduce cerebral edema.

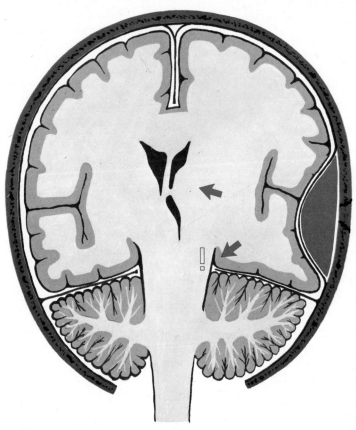

FIG. 70.—Epidural hematomas accumulate within hours of a head injury, through rupture of the middle meningeal artery— usually following skull fracture (which may not be visible). The hematoma displaces the dura from the inner table of the calvarium and compresses the brain. Clouding of consciousness, contralateral pyramidal signs and ipsilateral pupillary dilatation are warning signs. In the presence of midbrain compression (coma, tetraspasticity, dilated pupils), surgical evacuation may be too late.

Etiology: By rupture of the middle meningeal artery or one of its branches, even a small fracture of the calvarium may produce hemorrhage in the epidural space, i.e., between the inner table of the skull and dura. The dura is displaced inwardly by the hematoma, which compresses the underlying brain substance. Tentorial herniation and a decerebrate state may rapidly ensue.

Clinical: The circumstances often suggest a mild head injury. After a brief period of unconsciousness, the patient awakens; frequently he is discharged. Then, a few hours later ("lucid interval"), his level of consciousness begins to deteriorate, a pupil (usually ipsilateral) dilates and a hemiparesis appears. Signs of midbrain involvement follow promptly—nonreacting pupils, bilateral pyramidal signs, unconsciousness and extensor spasms. Pyrexia, tachycardia and raised blood pressure levels presage autonomic failure. The patient dies in coma.

Diagnosis: Skull roentgenograms may show a fracture line. Massive displacement of the midline structures will be revealed by CT scanning, carotid angiography (often essential to reveal the nature and extent of the lesion) and echoencephalography ("hematoma echo"). Electroencephalography (superfluous here) may show low-amplitude waves on the side of the hematoma. Life-threatening situation!

Treatment: Every minute is valuable as regards opening the skull and evacuating the hematoma. Prompt and continuous observations are required with respect to body temperature (hypothermia), pulse and blood pressure (cardiac and circulatory failure). Combat cerebral edema with attention to fluid and electrolyte balance (hematocrit? Na, K, Cl, Ca values?). In respiratory depression, intubation and artificial respiration are required as well as frequent aspiration of the bronchial tree. Antibiotics to prevent infection, gastric feeding.

SUBDURAL HEMATOMA (see Fig. 69, p. 162)

Rupture of bridging veins following microtrauma (advanced age, *anticoagulant therapy*, etc. may be predisposing factors) leads to subdural oozing, which may be bilateral. The hematoma presents as a chronic space-occupying intracranial lesion. The interval between the injury and the occurrence of symptoms and signs may be days, weeks or months. Prompt evacuation is essential.

Local Signs and Symptoms of Brain Tumors

Exceptionally as distant effects!

Frontal Lobe
Increased (reduced) drive
Personality change
Critical faculty reduced
Contralateral grasp reflex
also: Frontal ataxia
      Unilateral anosmia
      Deviation of the head to
        the side of the lesion
      Optic atrophy
      Broca's aphasia (Area 44)
      Hemiparesis

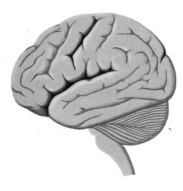

Paracentral lobule
   Bladder disturbances (see
   also p. 96)

Temporal Lobe
Auditory hallucinations
Wernicke's aphasia, amusia
Dreamy states
Uncinate fits

Parietal Lobe
Dominant hemisphere:
   Apraxia, agraphia, alexia,
   finger agnosia, acalculia,
   right/left confusion

Nondominant hemisphere:
   Constructive apraxia,
   contralateral neglect,
   dressing apraxia, anosognosia,
   spatial disorientation
   (drawing a map)
Bilateral:
   Hemihypesthesia, sensory
   (jacksonian) epilepsy

Occipital Lobe
Contralateral (homonymous)
   hemianopia, visual aura
   before seizures
Visual hallucinations
Difficulty recalling colors and
   faces (areas 18 and 19)

Brain Tumors

One to 2% of the population suffer and die from brain tumors. All neoplastic processes within the cranial cavity are grouped together under this heading, despite the fact that only a proportion arise from the brain substance itself (glial tumors). Tumors of the covering of the brain (meningiomas) and cerebral metastases produce a clinical picture similar to that produced by gliomas and glioblastomas.

If all intracranial tumors are regarded as a single entity, three clinical states can be defined: the *first stage* is asymptomatic. Occasionally, brain tumors are discovered as incidental findings at autopsy. An early symptom is epileptic seizures (epilepsy). Focal seizures always should raise the suspicion of an early brain tumor, as should adult-onset generalized seizures occurring without a previous history of seizure. Similarly, any focal neurologic sign, especially if slowly progressive, should prompt this diagnosis: weakness, sensory disturbances (even of sudden onset), homonymous and quadrantic hemianopia, cranial nerve palsies, alphasia, apraxia, agnosia.

The *intermediate stage* is characterized, apart from the focal epilepsy of the initial stage, by pressure on adjacent structures. The clinical picture now is reinforced by definite signs and symptoms of frontal, parietal, occipital or temporal lobe involvement. Hemiparesis is common: the patient experiences well-localized headaches. During this stage, the diagnosis can be made on the basis of the clinical findings, EEG, ultrasound (displacement of midline echo), brain scanning (CT or radioisotope imaging) or cerebral angiography. Skull roentgenograms may reveal pathologic calcification or a focal abnormality of the calvarium. The pituitary fossa may be destroyed and the dorsum sellae decalcified. In the *final or terminal stage*, signs and symptoms of raised intracranial pressure appear: papilledema, clouding of consciousness, vomiting, brain stem signs and coma. Lifesaving neurosurgical measures now are too late. Cerebral edema may develop in the parenchyma adjacent to the tumor and contribute to the neurologic symptoms and signs.

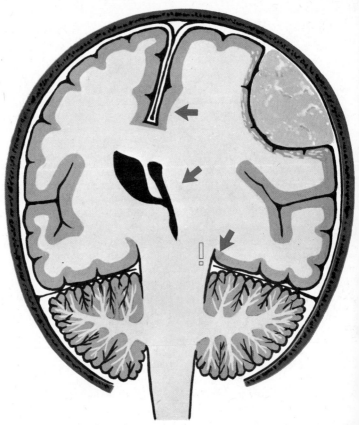

FIG. 71.—Meningiomas commonly are located over the convexity. They exert a space-occupying effect but do not inflltrate the brain. They cause focal irritation of the cortex (jacksonian attacks), compression of the ventricular system and—relatively late—raised intracranial pressure: mental changes, later clouding of consciousness, finally unconsciousness. Less amenable to successful surgery are parasagittal or falx, intraventricular (rare) or basilar meningiomas (arising from the base of the skull). Blood supply is frequently from the external carotid artery. Cerebral arteriography reveals a characteristic tumor stem.

Meningiomas

Ten to 20% of all brain tumors are *meningiomas*, i.e., neoplasms of the meninges. They occur most commonly in subjects aged 45–50 years and only rarely below 18 and above 70 years. Depending on the predominance of endothelial-like cells, fibrocytes or blood vessels within them, meningiomas are classified as *endotheliomatous, fibroblastic and angioblastic* in type. The endotheliomatous variety may consist of concentric layers that contain calcium deposits—so-called psammoma bodies. As the tumor expands, it displaces adjacent brain tissue. Angiography may reveal a typical and recognizable staining pattern, as well as an hypertrophied middle meningeal artery. Without operation, meningioma patients survive for 3–10 years. Complete removal is sometimes possible without damage to underlying cerebral tissue. Meningiomas tend to recur.

Clinical: Focal seizures may be the presenting feature. The site of the meningioma is crucial, and the following are distinguished: *convexity meningiomas* (over all lobes), which lead to focal disturbances of higher cortical function; *sphenoid wing meningiomas*, which produce an upper cranial nerve syndrome (3rd–6th cranial nerves and exophthalmos); *olfactory groove meningiomas* (anosmia); *tuberculum sellae meningiomas* (visual field defects due to pressure on the optic nerve); *tentorial meningioma* (often "hourglass" shape, with supra- *and* infratentorial symptoms and signs); *falx and parasagittal meningiomas* (few typical clinical features). Weakness seldom is marked, and papilledema occurs late—as do all the neurologic signs. Similarly, the EEG changes are minimal, producing nonspecific features and some asymmetry. Echoencephalography may show significant lateral displacement of the midline echo. Carotid angiography provides a specific diagnosis if the characteristic tumor stain is present (no early venous filling). Lumbar puncture is absolutely contraindicated in the later stages; earlier, the protein content often is increased.

Differential Diagnosis: Other chronic space-occupying intracranial masses.

Treatment: Surgical excision. Control edema. Subsequently, symptomatic epilepsy is common.

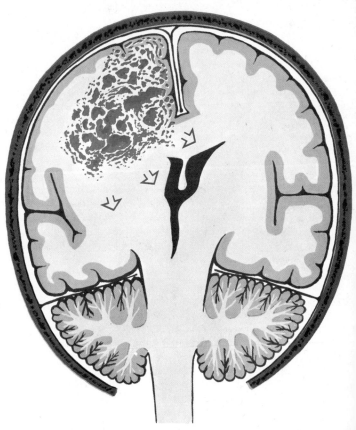

Fɪɢ. 72.—Hemorrhagic glioblastoma infiltrating the brain and spreading into the opposite hemisphere via the corpus callosum. The ventricular system is less markedly displaced and the cerebral cortex not as severely damaged as in meningiomas. The neurologic deficits are more marked, but the seizures are frequently less focal in nature. Gliomas have a poorly defined margin and may contain calcium deposits (oligodendroglioma) or cystic areas (astrocytoma).

GLIOMAS AND GLIOBLASTOMAS

Ten to 15% of all brain tumors are gliomas (those arising from astrocytes = astrocytomas and those from oligodendrocytes = oligodendrogliomas). These primary brain tumors expand slowly by infiltration, usually occurring in subjects between 25 and 45 years of age or more; they are common in the elderly and very rare in children. For several years they may run an almost asymptomatic course. The rarest types are the *ependymomas* (arising from ependymal cells, 1–4%) and the *spongioblastomas* (arising from spongioblasts, 2–7%)—which grow faster and usually appear more malignant clinically. All gliomas may undergo malignant degeneration, and various forms transitional to the common malignant tumor, the *glioblastoma* (13–20% of all tumors), are seen. Glioblastomas generally occur between 40 and 60 years but may be seen throughout adulthood; they are more common in men (2:1) and very rare in children and elderly subjects. On histologic examination the tumor shows a bizarre pattern: foci of necrosis and hemorrhage are common. The clinical course, from the time of the evident symptomatology to death, is measured in months.

Clinical: Gliomas and glioblastomas give rise to more evident signs of cerebral involvement than do meningiomas. Gliomas show a slowly progressive parade of symptoms. Dramatic episodes may be heralded by focal or generalized seizures. Glioblastomas may appear suddenly—through hemorrhage into the tumor. The neurologic deficits and the impairment of higher cortical function indicate the location of the lesion. Nonspecific mental disturbances are common (mild intellectual impairment or personality change—"tumor psyche"). Loss of initiative or affect and lact of interest often are the presenting symptoms. The diagnosis of avascular gliomas may be difficult by angiography but glioblastomas show irregularly dilated blood vessels and early venous filling. CT scanning reveals the extent of the tumor and the surrounding edema accurately but does not permit differentiation from metastatic deposits. Echoencephalography reveals only a midline shift and the EEG shows a focal abnormality.

Treatment: Surgical excision (as radical as possible) followed by whole-brain radiation therapy and chemotherapy.

Incidence of Individual Tumor Types
(Arteriovenous Malformations)*

Frontal Lobe

Meningioma	31%
Glioblastoma	19%
Astrocytoma	17%
Oligodendroglioma	16%
Metastasis	5%
Ependymoma	1%

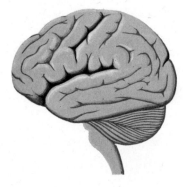

Parietal Lobe

Meningioma	31%
Glioblastoma	22%
Astrocytoma	12%
Oligodendroglioma	9%
Ependymoma	7.5%
Metastasis	5%
Arteriovenous mal- formation	3%

Occipital Lobe

Meningioma	27%
Glioblastoma	26%
Arteriovenous mal- formation	9%
Astrocytoma	7%
Ependymoma	7%
Metastasis	7%
Oligodendroglioma	5%
Spongioblastoma	4%

Temporal Lobe

Glioblastoma	29%
Meningioma	26%
Oligodendroglioma	12%
Astrocytoma	12%
Metastasis	3%
Ependymoma	2%
Arteriovenous mal- formation	1%

Brainstem

Glioblastoma	53%
Oligodendroglioma	13%
Astrocytoma	10%
Metastasis	6%
Spongioblastoma	2%
Arteriovenous mal- formation	2%
Meningioma	1%

*after Zulch

Cerebral metastases are very common. In bronchial carcinomas (over 50% of all metastases), the patient's presenting symptoms may refer to the intracranial metastases rather than the primary tumor. However, breast cancer (9%), hypernephroma (about 5%), uterine (3%), rectal (2.5%) and prostatic cancer (2%) (data from Scheid) tend to develop pulmonary metastases ("lung filter") before brain metastases. In any subject over 45 years with raised intracranial pressure—but also in younger subjects—the diagnosis of metastases should be considered. A chest roentgenogram is part of the diagnostic procedure for patients with brain tumors.

Clinical: Apart from hemispheric or brain stem lesions, which present a focal clinical picture, severe and explicable organic brain syndromes occur. Epileptiform seizures are common. Often attacks of mild derangement lead to symptomatic psychoses or increasing clouding of consciousness, with a variable pattern of focal features. Electroencephalography may show two or more focal abnormalities (intermittent or delta wave foci). Patients in whom clinical localization is poor or impossible usually harbor multiple metastases. Cerebral angiography reveals either areas of neovascularization or avascular masses. CT and radioisotope imaging of the brain probably are more suitable investigative methods, the first named being the most accurate. Echoencephalography not invariably shows midline displacement.

Treatment: Surgical excision should be considered in solitary metastases. Palliation of symptoms can be achieved by cranial irradiation and high-dose corticosteroids.

Intraventricular tumors such as *choroid plexus papillomas*, pinealomas (aqueductal occlusion, precocious puberty) and *epidermoids, dermoids and teratomas* are less common.

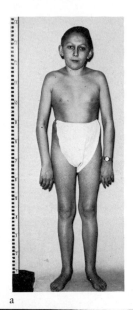

a

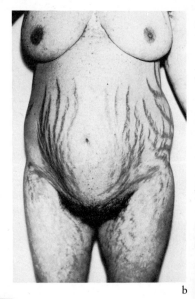

b

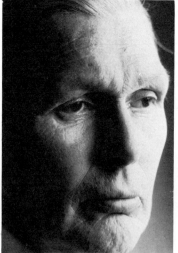

c

FIG. 73.—(a) Craniopharyngioma. A 25-year-old-man with short stature and lack of secondary sex characteristics. (b) Basophilic pituitary adenoma (Cushing's disease). Truncal obesity with red striae, secondary amenorrhea (impotence), osteoporosis, hyperglycemia, hypocalcemia and low eosinophil counts. (c) Chromophobe adenoma with panhypopituitarism. Loss of facial hair and fine wrinkles in the skin.

174

Suprasellar Tumors, Pituitary Adenomas

CRANIOPHARYNGIOMAS

Craniopharyngiomas are the most frequent suprasellar tumors, comprising 3% of all intracranial tumors. They are derived from Rathke's pouch, grow very slowly, compressing and displacing the optic chiasm rostrally, the third ventricle superiorly, and the hypophysis ventrally. Microscopic features consist of cords or sheets of epithelial cells arranged in several layers, which are separated by loose connective tissue. Complete surgical removal often is technically difficult and recurrences are common.

Clinically, there are endocrinologic abnormalities—amenorrhea, disturbances in growth (growth failure in children), hyperthermia, optic nerve atrophy, and raised intracranial pressure due to obstruction of the interventricular foramen. Plain skull films show suprasellar calcifications and atrophy of the dorsum sellae.

PITUITARY ADENOMAS

These are tumors of adults, occurring most frequently between 37 to 41 years of age. Their intrasellar expansile growth leads to ballooning of the sella with later destruction of the dorsum and floor of the sella turcica. Extrasellar extension endangers the optic nerve and chiasm leading to bitemporal hemianopia and loss of vision. Inferior extension through the floor of the sella may predispose to ascending infections (meningitis). About three-fourths of all pituitary adenomas *(chromophobe adenomas)* lead to panhypopituitarism— secondary amenorrhea, hypothyroidism, hypotension and diabetes mellitus. Prolactin secreting adenomas frequently present with amenorrhea and galactorrhea. Sudden clinical deterioration with clouding of consciousness, diplopia, failure of vision can develop due to spontaneous hemorrhage into the tumor (pituitary apoplexy). Suprasellar extension is an operative indication to preserve vision. A transsphenoidal approach has led to good surgical results. In these cases hormonal substitution therapy (thyroxin, corticosteroids) may not even be necessary. The eosinophilic adenoma leads to gigantism or acromegaly (enlargement of feet and hands), hypertension, diabetes mellitus and headaches. The basophilic adenoma (Cushing's disease) is rare.

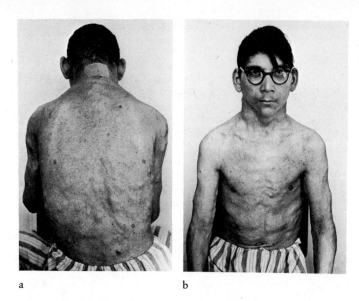

a   b

FIG. 74.—von Recklinghausen's neurofibromatosis. Multiple
café au lait spots and numerous subcutaneous neurofibromas are
scattered over the trunk of this patient. Neck shows large nodular
neurofibromas. Multiple nerve root neurofibromas lead to spinal
cord compression.

Phakomatoses are a group of diseases that have in common developmental neuroectodermal dysplastic processes which affect the skin, the nervous system or the eyes. During life these distinctive malformations enlarge to multiple tumors affecting the involved organs. Within this group are included:

Von Recklinghausen's neurofibromatosis: This is a frequent familial disorder (1:2000) of dominant inheritance. Pigmentary nevi and café-au-lait spots of the skin are associated with multiple subcutaneous neurofibromas, neurofibromas of cranial nerves and nerve roots. Involvement of cranial nerves in particular gives rise to bilateral acoustic schwannomas. Nerve root neurofibromas may lead to segmental deficits and spinal cord compression.

Tuberose sclerosis (Bourneville's disease): This autosomal dominant condition is characterized by angiofibromas (adenoma sebaceum) involving the face in a butterfly distribution. Glial nodules, containing spongioblast-like cells, may affect the retina (blindness), the cerebral cortex and subependymal layers and lead to focal seizures and obstruction of the foramen of Monroe and the cerebral aqueduct. Hemiparesis, tetraparesis and mental retardation are frequent. Associated visceral tumors include rhabdomyosarcomas of the heart and mixed neoplasms of the kidney.

Von Hippel-Lindau's disease (retinocerebellar angiomatosis): This familial disease is characterized by multiple hemangioblastomas localized most frequently to the retina and cerebellum, less often to the spinal cord. The small hemangioblastomas of the cerebellum have a tendency to develop large cysts.

Sturge-Weber's disease (encephalotrigeminal angiomatosis): Here there is an extensive unilateral cutaneous angioma of the face involving the territory of the first and second, seldom the third, division of the trigeminal nerve. The associated cerebral involvement consists of a leptomeningeal encephalic angiomatosis accompanied by alterations in the underlying cortex (gliosis and parallel linear calcifications). Seizures and mental retardation are frequent.

Therapy: Symptomatic tumors require surgical resection.

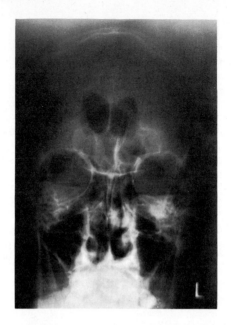

Fig. 75.—Pneumoencephalogram (PEG) showing characteristic features of cerebral atrophy. Dilatation of the ventricular system and profuse accumulation of air in the convexity sulci (sulcal air not visible in this illustration).

DIFFERENTIAL DIAGNOSIS OF CEREBRAL ATROPHY AND ATROPHIC PROCESSES DUE TO OTHER CAUSES

Clinical: Slow, steady progression—not stuttering course as in cerebrovascular disease (commonly), disseminated encephalomyelitis or microhemorrhages into a glioblastoma. Focal neurologic findings transient or absent.

Investigations: Echo-EEG reveals a widened but centrally located third ventricle. EEG: predominance of fast, low-voltage bursts, no lateralizing features. CSF: usually only an increased protein content, no inflammatory changes (which may be present in general paresis). PEG: widening of ventricular system and gross pooling of air over the cerebral convexities. Lateral ventricles widened.

Other: Laboratory results usually normal. Attention should be paid to the family history.

178

Cerebral Atrophy

Etiology: Many diseases lead to atrophic brain lesions with ganglion cell degeneration and glial proliferation. One group of such diseases are those commencing in middle or advanced age, which are slowly progressive and eventually lead to generalized cerebral atrophy. Other similar diseases include the following: systemic medical disorders, e.g., liver disease, toxic and other nutritional diseases (alcohol and early malnutrition—specifically protein deficiency), atypical trauma, e.g., the punch-drunk syndrome of boxers (so-called *dementia pugilistica*) and genetic factors (*Alzheimer's disease:* dominant or recessive, *Pick's disease:* dominant or polygenic). There is hydrocephalus ex vacua and asternal dilatation; microscopically one sees ganglion cell loss and Alzheimer's neurofibrillary tangles.

Clinical: All types show psychopathologic changes such as diminished awareness, blunting or disintegration of affect, deficient thought and memory processes and loss of drive. Pick's disease may appear as early as the third decade of life: characteristically in this disease, relatively circumscribed parts of the cerebral hemispheres undergo atrophy. Personality changes precede the dementia: amnestic aphasia, echolalia, palililia, logorrhea and an asymbolism may be present. The average duration of this fatal disease is about 7 years.

Alzheimer's disease commences in the fifth or sixth decade and the victims survive an average of 7 years. The patient's intellectual ability deteriorates early: signs of aphasia, apraxia, agnosia, and logospasm seldom are absent. The patient's inactivity or episodes of agitation may be clinically prominent. In the final stages some, but not all, patients tend to waste away. As in Pick's disease, circumscribed foci of atrophy can be demonstrated—in contrast to senile dementia, which appears only around the 70th year and which may be heralded by delusions.

Treatment: No specific therapy so far known.

International Classification of Epileptic Seizures*

I.   Partial Seizures (seizures beginning locally)
    A. Partial seizures with elementary symptomatology (generally
       without impairment of consciousness).
       1. With motor symptoms [includes Jacksonian seizures]
       2. With special sensory or somatosensory symptoms
       3. With autonomic symptoms
       4. Compound forms
    B. Partial seizures with complex symptomatology (generally
       with impairment of consciousness).
       [temporal lobe or psychomotor seizures]
       1. With impairment of consciousness only
       2. With cognitive symptomatology
       3. With affective symptomatology
       4. With "psychosensory" symptomatology
       5. With "psychomotor" symptomatology (automatisms)
       6. Compound forms
    C. Partial seizures secondarily generalized
II. Generalized Seizures (bilaterally symmetrical and without local
    onset)
       1. Absences [petit mal]
       2. Bilateral massive epileptic myoclonus
       3. Infantile spasms
       4. Clonic seizures
       5. Tonic seizures
       6. Tonic-clonic seizures [grand mal]
       7. Atonic seizures
       8. Akinetic seizures
III. Unilateral Seizures (or predominantly)
IV. Unclassified Epileptic Seizures (due to incomplete data)

*Abstracted from Gastaut, H. Clinical and electroencephalographical classification
of epileptic seizures. Epilepsia 11: 102-113, 1970)

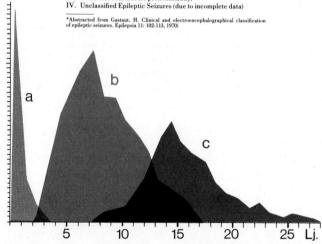

Fig. 76.—Many seizures are age dependent (adapted from Janz).
(a) Infantile spasms are seen only in the first two years of life. *(b)*
Typical absence or petit mal seizures occur almost exclusively in
childhood between 2 and 17 years, with a peak frequency at about
8 years. *(c)* Myoclonic seizures are seen between 8 to 27 years with a
peak around 14 years. Typical grand mal seizures are seen most
frequently in adulthood.

180

Epilepsy and Other Seizure Disorders (see also p. 28f)

Etiology: Seizures are a reaction of the brain or a specific part of the brain to numerous types of trauma. Certain drugs (Metrazol, Bemegride, etc.) and electroshock therapy provoke epileptiform attacks. Generalized convulsions occur as a result of inflammatory processes (meningitis) or cerebrovascular lesions, as an early sign of brain tumors, toxins (alcohol), metabolic-nutritional disturbances and the effects of trauma to the brain. Early traumatic epilepsy, i.e., an attack occurring within a few hours of the accident, has a good prognosis; *late traumatic epilepsy* is due to brain scarring (dural scar) and appears many months or years after the accident. (*Epilepsy* frequently is the result of brain damage in early life (pre-, peri- or postnatal)—asphyxia, intracranial hematomas, kernicterus, postinflammatory scarring (meningitis, encephalitis). These seizures with a known organic or metabolic substrate are best termed symptomatic epilepsies.

In other cases, epileptiform seizures may be encountered in families in which no demonstrable organic cause of the attacks can be demonstrated. Here, the term *idiopathic generalized epilepsy* is used. Frequently the question of whether a definable organic process or a genetic defect is the root cause remains unanswered in an individual patient. In many cases, both factors contribute.

Any individual, under particular circumstances, may suffer an epileptic seizure. Close to 1% of the population of the United States has epilepsy. A variety of situations may underlie the individual attack: apart from residual scarring and a propensity to epilepsy, incidental factors such as febrile illnesses, lack of sleep, alcohol, etc. play a part.

Clinical: The most important sign (but not the only one) is the attack. The most dangerous type is the generalized convulsion (grand mal), which may cause damage to the brain and other parts of the body. The aura, the tonic contractions and the succeeding clonic phase are typical, followed by the postictal sleep. An attack is recognized by skin abrasions, fecal and urinary incontinence and tongue biting—although these signs need not accompany each attack.

A Guide to the Etiologic Differential Diagnosis of Epilepsy

Generalized Seizures: (Try to rule out secondary variety!)

Often cryptogenic (leads to nocturnal attacks): "genuine," familial.

Or expression of generalized brain damage: effect of drugs, alcohol (withdrawal), hypoglycemia, diffuse organic brain lesion.

Focal Attacks: (Try to exclude secondary focalization from primary generalized epilepsy!)

a. Result of brain damage in early life: Was the mother ill during pregnancy? Placental anomalies at birth? Fetal erythroblastosis with jaundice? Meningitides or encephalitides in early childhood?

Later criteria: motor retardation. Spasticity (cerebral palsy), intellectual deterioration—IQ 50–69, i.e., analogous to mental age: 8–12. Debility—IQ 20–49, i.e., analogous to mental age: 3–7. Imbecility—IQ 0–19 (sometimes impossible to asses), i.e., analogous to mental age: 0–2. = idiocy.

b. Results of craniocerebral trauma: previous contusion or dural scar with neurologic, psychopathologic, EEG or CT-scan abnormalities?

c. Inflammatory lesions: brain abscess, granulomatous encephalitis, adhesive arachnoiditis? ESR, hemogram, increased CSF protein or cell content, etc.?

d. Brain tumor (metastases?): focal neurologic signs? Disturbances of higher cortical function? "Tumor psychosis" computerized tomography, echo- and electroencephalographic and scintigraphic findings? Chest roentgenogram?

e. Cerebrovascular lesion: risk factors—hypercholesterolemia, arterial hypertension, diabetes? Pregnancy (dural venous sinus thrombosis), cardiac defects, postmyocardial infarction syndrome (embolism)?

f. Degenerative atrophic cerebral lesions, inborn errors of metabolism? Attacks that occur only in the morning (waking epilepsy) are typical of symptomatic epilepsy.

Each seizure favors the onset of another; it lowers the seizure threshold. In this way, *status epilepticus* develops, which is defined as the occurrence of at least three, but often multiple, attacks succeeding one and other without regaining total consciousness and which may be fatal because of exhaustion, cerebral edema or other complications (cardiac arrest, pneumonia).

Many epileptic variants exist: in *focal seizures*, discharges from the underlying epileptic focus may provoke a variety of sensory and motor deficits. Of great importance in the history are details of the aura. Such focal attacks may also occur after many years of idiopathic generalized epilepsy as a result of concomitant ganglion cell degeneration (trauma, seizure-induced anoxia).

Nonconvulsive attacks are common in children: Infantile spasms are characterized by "jackknifing and saalam attacks." In early school age, petit mal is a brief absence with impairment of consciousness and associated classical EEG findings (generalized 3/sec spike and wave pattern); at the time of puberty myoclonic jerks are often seen.

Psychomotor attacks with clouding of consciousness (dream states) may last for many minutes. The patient may be able to carry out simple commands and even utter intelligible words, but his behavior is aimless, his thought processes incoherent, and he may execute strange movements. He fails to react—or reacts inadequately—to his environment, and subsequently exhibits a postictal amnesia. If the attack lasts longer—hours or days, sometimes weeks—the descriptive term *"dream state"* is used. The patient's atypical behavior may lead to criminal acts, for which he is not responsible. Medicolegally, each individual incident must be investigated and proved. Epileptic equivalents represent episodically occurring states of depression, irritability, obsessional agitation and occasionally delusions.

Symptomatic psychoses with hallucinations may develop. These psychoses may occur at a time when the patient's seizures are well controlled.

Epileptics should not drive motor vehicles!

ADVICE ON THE TREATMENT OF EPILEPSY

Status Epilepticus (Life-threatening!)
1. Phenytoin 1000 mg (12–15 mg/kg) i.v. at a rate of 50 mg/min
2. Phenobarbital 100–300 mg i.v. or i.m., followed by 4 mg/kg i.m. at 2–6 hour intervals (Total dose 500 mg)
3. Diazepam, usually 50–10 mg i.v. (Danger: Apnea!)
4. General anesthesia
   Blood pressure, respiratory rate and ECG are monitored. Rule out acute electrolyte imbalance (hyponatremia) and hypoglycemia.

Grand Mal
   Drug of choice: Phenytoin (Dilantin). Adjust dosage to obtain phenytoin serum levels of 10–20 μg/ml. Usual maintenance dose: 300 mg daily, or phenytoin plus phenobarbital (Luminal), or phenytoin plus primidone (Mysoline)

Focal seizures with complex symptomatology (psychomotor)
   Phenytoin, or combination of phenytoin and primidone, phenytoin and carbamazepine (Tegretol), or phenytoin plus primidone plus carbamazepine

Focal seizures with elementary symptomatology
   (as under focal seizures with complex symptomatology above)

Petit Mal
   Ethosuximinide (Zarontin), or Clonazepam (Clonopin), or sodium valproate (Depakene). Concomitant use of phenytoin or phenobarbitol is often necessary to control associated grand mal convulsions.

Infantile spasms
   ACTH, or dexamethasone
   Clonazepam (Clonopin)
   Watch for idiosyncratic side effects: blood dyscrasias, dermatitis, lupus-like syndrome—and toxicity: nystagmus, ataxia, sedation, polyneuropathy. Treatment always must be tailored to the patient and administered under EEG control!

Epileptic personality changes develop as a result of repeated brain damage caused by numerous epileptic attacks, perhaps also because of psychopathologic equivalents, which are the basis of the attacks—fussiness, moodiness, irritability, an unusual "viscosity" of affect, a slowness in thought processes and a pedantic attitude toward life and perseverance.

Diagnosis: Essential for the diagnosis is the epileptiform seizure, properly observed and described. Each detail may provide important clues as to the etiology or localization of the underlying lesion. Nearly as useful in diagnosis are the EEG findings, revealing paroxysmal features which are specific or suspicious of epilepsy. However, paroxysmal potentials are not present in every EEG tracing: many electrical leads may be required or special provocation (sleep deprivation, sleep EEG, photic stimulation, etc.) to elicit the typical EEG findings, and sometimes these are completely absent. Relatives of epileptics may have EEG tracings exhibiting paroxysmal features without having experienced attacks themselves. It is most important to distinguish primary idiopathic epilepsy from symptomatic seizures caused by space-occupying intracranial lesions—only after 2–10 years can a tumor be totally excluded as a cause of epilepsy. Therefore, if the attacks are focal in character, neuroradiologic investigations (CT scan, cerebral angiography) are essential, and these may have to be repeated at intervals to define the nature of the underlying process. A significant proportion of brain tumors—also abscesses, etc.—first manifest themselves clinically as epileptic attacks. Remember hypoglycemia and uremia!

Treatment: The cause (i.e., the nature of the epileptogenic focus) must be determined, and corrected, if possible. Often this is impossible. Second, anticonvulsants must be used to raise the seizure threshold (generalized, simple focal and psychomotor seizures: phenytoin, phenobarbital, mysoline, carbamazepine. Petit mal: Ethosuximide, clonazepam, sodium valproate). Contributing factors must be eliminated (forbid alcohol, recommend plenty of sleep).

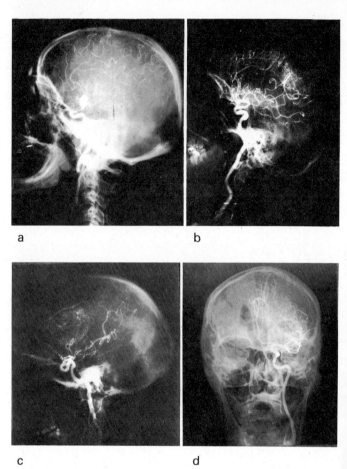

Fig. 77.—Four important causes of headache: **(a)** Aneurysm of anterior communicating artery. **(b)** Meningioma of the parietal convexity. **(c)** Frontocentral glioblastoma multiforme. **(d)** Extensive right subdural hematoma.

Headache, Facial Pain

Headaches are one of the most common neurologic complaints. They may be a symptom of brain, scalp or cranial nerve disease. Details of their frequency and duration are important. *Migraine,* which almost invariably is familial, appears in attacks that are unilateral or bilateral in their distribution; in a previously well subject, severe headache develops within 1–2 hours, usually more promptly. In two-thirds of sufferers, the headache is accompanied by nausea and vomiting (Heyck), and it recurs periodically. The pain has a throbbing or hammering character, and pallor or fortification spectra may be associated with it—also transient speech disturbances and sensory or motor deficits—*migrain accompagnée.* The diagnosis is justified only if these criteria are present and if an organic cerebral lesion can be excluded. The cause is thought to be a vascular hyperreactivity of extracerebral and cerebral vessels. Particular personality traits are recognizable in many migraine sufferers, which are only partly a result of this disease. Ambition, intolerance, a tendency to aggressive behavior and personal insecurity are prominent. The actual attack lasts hours or days. Tachycardia, dryness of the mouth, diarrhea and polyuria may occur. Ergotamines are particularly useful in treatment.

Vasomotor headache reflects vascular-induced autonomic dysregulation caused by fatigue, alcoholic "hangover," mental stress, other disturbances of the sleep/wake cycle and intracranial lesions. Drug abuse or even a regular intake of analgesics and excessive nicotine or caffeine ingestion aggravates autonomic dysregulation and thereby provokes vasomotor headaches. Many patients in the course of weeks or months embark on a vicious circle, since the transient pain-killing properties of analgesics may aggravate the underlying disease.

Numerous intracranial diseases begin with headache. However, this feature seldom is significant diagnostically, since the patient may pay little or no attention to it. Sometimes he admits to headache only after specific questioning.

REVIEW OF FACIAL NEURALGIAS		
Name	*Pain Distribution*	*Trigger Zone*
Trigeminal neuralgia	Upper and lower jaws, in distribution of 2d and 3d divisions of trigeminal n.	Mouth, and trunks of infraorbital and mental nerves
Auriculotemporal neuralgia	Temple and auricular area, "gustatory sweating"	Act of chewing
Nasociliary (Trélat-Charlin's) neuralgia	Globe and inner canthus of eye, nasal region and lacrimal apparatus	Act of chewing, canthus of eye
Pterygopalatine ganglion (Sluder's) neuralgia	Orbits and nasal region; Often chronic	Sneezing
Intermedius neuralgia (Ramsay Hunt's syndrome)	Auditory canal and inner ear; herpetic, vesicular eruption in auditory canal	
Glossopharyngeal neuralgia	Tongue, auditory canal and inner ear	Surface of tongue, gums (act of swallowing)
Superior laryngeal neuralgia (Avellis's syndrome)	Larynx, surface of tongue, epiglottis	Swallowing, speaking, coughing, yawning

In a typical case of facial neuralgia, the attacks of pain are paroxysmal and may last only a few seconds.

Always exclude a local cause: seek ophthalmologic, otologic and dental advice. However, if no local cause is identified, *treatment* should be supervised by a neurologist. The attacks may be suppressed with phenytoin or Tegretol, and the limbic system (reaction to pain) suppressed by means of ataractics and neuroleptics (combination of imipramine and neuroleptic, i.e., Triavil). (See also Heyck, *Headache*, Thieme, Stuttgart, 1969).

Headaches are frequent complaints if the patient's affective threshold is seriously altered—thus, in the *crises of everday life*, in *abnormal (neurotic) situations* and in *endogenous depression*. Also, stress situations may lead to chronic "tension" headaches.

Numerous generalized diseases cause headache, especially *arterial hypertension* (*pheochromocytoma* should be considered in paroxysmal attacks), *azotemia* due to renal insufficiency, *hypotension*, blood disorders, such as anemia, *leukemia, polycythemia, diabetes mellitus* and *hypoglycemia*, and various *intoxications*.

Hypertensive encephalopathy, often accompanied by hyaline degeneration of small arteries with microscopic *hemorrhages* and local transudates and cerebral edema may be responsible for transient neurologic deficits (transient attacks of weakness, aphasia, apraxia, agnosia) and psychopathologic features (mental clouding) as well as headache.

Brief (15–30 minutes) and very intense headaches are found in *cluster headaches* (Bing-Horton syndrome, histamine cephalalgia). The attacks usually occur at night, often after drinking alcohol, and the headache is preceded by the development of a painful parietal or frontal scalp. The pain, which may be sufficiently intense to prompt thoughts of suicide, responds well to ergotamines.

Giant cell arteritis may produce very severe headache if the disease process involves the superficial temporal artery. Other arteries may also be affected, including intracranial arteries *(Horton syndrome)*. The disease is heralded by inflammatory features (very high ESR), which are evident in the artery (histologic examination in longitudinal section) and which respond well to corticosteroids. If treatment is delayed, the ophthalmic artery may be affected, with the risk of blindness.

Headaches caused by disorders of the temporomandibular joints and inflammatory or neoplastic lesions of the paranasal sinuses must be treated by the appropriate physicians or surgeons.

Facial neuralgia, mentioned above, is characterized by attacks of intense pain that characteristically are short-lived (seconds) and tend to recur. It is found mainly in elderly subjects and often responds well to anticonvulsants (phenytoin, Tegretol). Occasionally patients are resistant to this treatment and neurosurgical measures (electrocoagulation of Gasserian ganglion) should be considered.

189

DIAGNOSTIC FLOWSHEET FOR THE MANAGEMENT OF HEADACHE

Examination	Conclusions
History:	
Accident?	Subdural hematoma?
Infections?	Meningitis, encephalitis?
Malignancy in other organs?	Metastases
Headaches for years	Migraine, vasomotor distur-
for weeks, months	bance?
for hours, days	Space-occupying lesion?
Location: unilateral	Meningitis, subarachnoid
occipital	hemorrhage?
	Migraine? Neoplasm?
	Meningitis, cervical spondylo-
	sis?
Duration of Pain Attacks:	
up to 5 minutes	Facial neuralgia (5th, 7th, 9th)?
up to 1 hour	Horton's disease
6 hours/days	Migraine
constant	"Habitual" vasomotor disease
	Organic intracranial lesion
Family History:	Migraine
Accompanying Symptoms	
transient	Migraine
lasting	Organic intracranial lesion
Neurologic Findings:	
Meningism	Meningitis, infratentorial
	mass lesion
Papilledema	Space-occupying lesion
Ocular palsies	Basal meningitis, space
	occupying lesion
Pyramidal tract signs	Hemispheric lesion
Mental Features:	
Increased pain threshold	Vasomotor headache, cervical
	syndrome
Roentgenograms:	
Paranasal sinuses	Sinusitis
"Pressure Sella," digital	
impressions	Space-occupying lesion

190

Calcification	Tumor, postinflammatory deposits
Pineal shift	Hematoma, tumor

Echoencephalography:
Displaced midline echo?   Unilateral hemispheric process

EEG:
| Focal findings? | Space-occupying process |
| Spikes, mild dysrhythmia | Migraine |

Scintigraphy:
Increased uptake?   Tumor, metastases, hematoma?

General Medical Conditions: Hypertension? Uremia? Liver Disease? Poisoning?

Only when indicated following physical examination:

CSF Examination:	*Carotid or Vertebral Angiography*
Turbidity, pleocytosis	
Uniformly blood stained xanthochromia	Meningitis
	Subarachnoid hemorrhage
	Occlusion, displacement, tumor stain, or vascular malformations

NARCOLEPSY

Patients with narcolepsy experience attacks of disturbed night sleep, hypnagogic hallucinations, sleep paralysis and a loss of muscle tone—during fright, anger and laughing (cataplexy, transient "laughing attack"). Narcolepsy may be idiopathic or follow encephalitis or cerebral hemochromatosis.

Therapeutic trial with methylphenidate (Ritelin). *Danger:* risk of habit formation! Cataplectic attacks frequently respond to tricyclic antidepressants (Imipramine).

Appendix

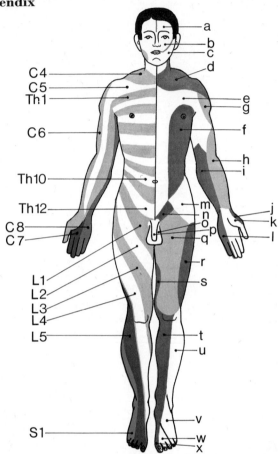

Fig. 78.—**Sensory Innervation:** *Frontal view. (a)* Frontal N. *(b)* Infraorbital N. *(c)* Mandibular N. *(d)* Supraclavicular N. *(e)* Anterior cutaneous rami. *(f)* Lateral cutaneous rami of intercostal N. *(g)* Axillary N. *(h)* Lateral antebrachial cutaneous N. (Forearm musculocutaneous N.) *(i)* Medial cutaneous N. of forearm. *(j)* Radial N. *(k)* Median N. *(l)* Ulnar N. *(m)* Iliohypogastric N. *(n)* Genitofemoral N. *(o)* Ilioinguinal N. *(p)* Dorsal N. of penis. *(q)* Femoral N. *(r)* Lateral femoral cutaneous N. *(s)* Obturator N. *(t)* Saphenous N. *(u)* Lateral sural cutaneous N. *(v)* Superficial peroneal N. *(w)* Deep peroneal N. *(x)* Tibial N.

192

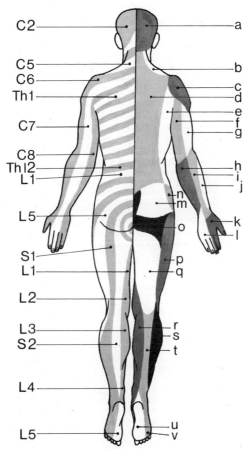

Fig. 79.—**Sensory Innervation:** *Posterior view. (a)* Occipital
N. *(b)* Supraclavicular N. *(c)* Axillary N. *(d)* Dorsal roots of cutaneous rami of intercostal N. *(e)* Lateral rami of intercostal N. *(f)* Medial brachial cutaneous N. *(g)* Posterior cutaneous N. of arm (from
radial N.). *(h)* Lateral sural cutaneous N. *(i)* Dorsal antebrachial
cutaneous N. (from radial N.) *(j)* Lateral antebrachial cutaneous N.
(from musculocutaneous N.) *(k)* Radial N. *(l)* Ulnar N. *(m)* Posteri-
or rami of upper lumbar N. *(n)* Iliohypogastric N. *(o)* Gluteral
branches of posterior femoral cutaneous N. *(p)* Lateral femoral
cutaneous N. *(q)* Posterior femoral cutaneous N. *(r)* Saphenous N.
(s) Lateral sural cutaneous N. *(t)* Sural N. *(u)* and *(v)* Medial and
lateral plantar N.

193

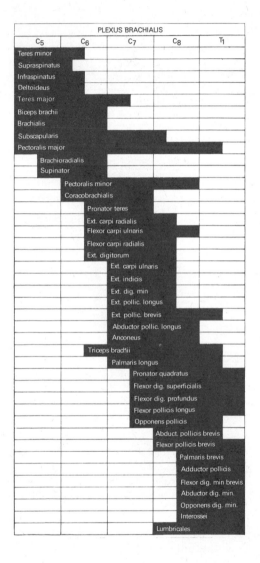

Fig. 80.—Segmental innervation of brachial plexus, supplying arm and shoulder muscles.

194

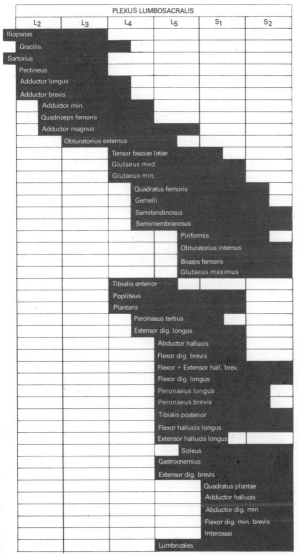

Fig. 81.—Segmental motor innervation of lumbosacral plexus, supplying muscles of pelvis and lower limbs.

195

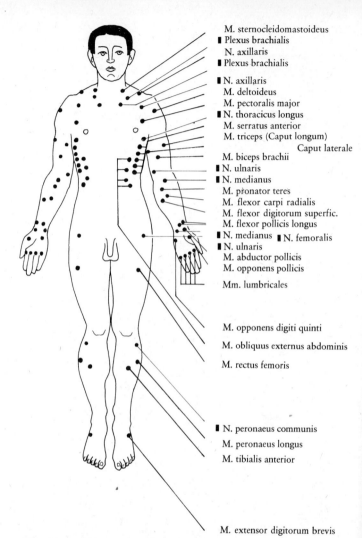

M. sternocleidomastoideus
▌Plexus brachialis
N. axillaris
▌Plexus brachialis

▌N. axillaris
M. deltoideus
M. pectoralis major
▌N. thoracicus longus
M. serratus anterior
M. triceps (Caput longum)
Caput laterale
M. biceps brachii
▌N. ulnaris
▌N. medianus
M. pronator teres
M. flexor carpi radialis
M. flexor digitorum superfic.
M. flexor pollicis longus
▌N. medianus ▌N. femoralis
▌N. ulnaris
M. abductor pollicis
M. opponens pollicis

Mm. lumbricales

M. opponens digiti quinti

M. obliquus externus abdominis

M. rectus femoris

▌N. peronaeus communis
M. peronaeus longus
M. tibialis anterior

M. extensor digitorum brevis

FIG. 82.—Points of stimulation of muscles and nerves. Frontal view. *Note:* these points vary from individual to individual, and may be shifted in the same individual in the presence of a lesion of the lower motoneuron.

196

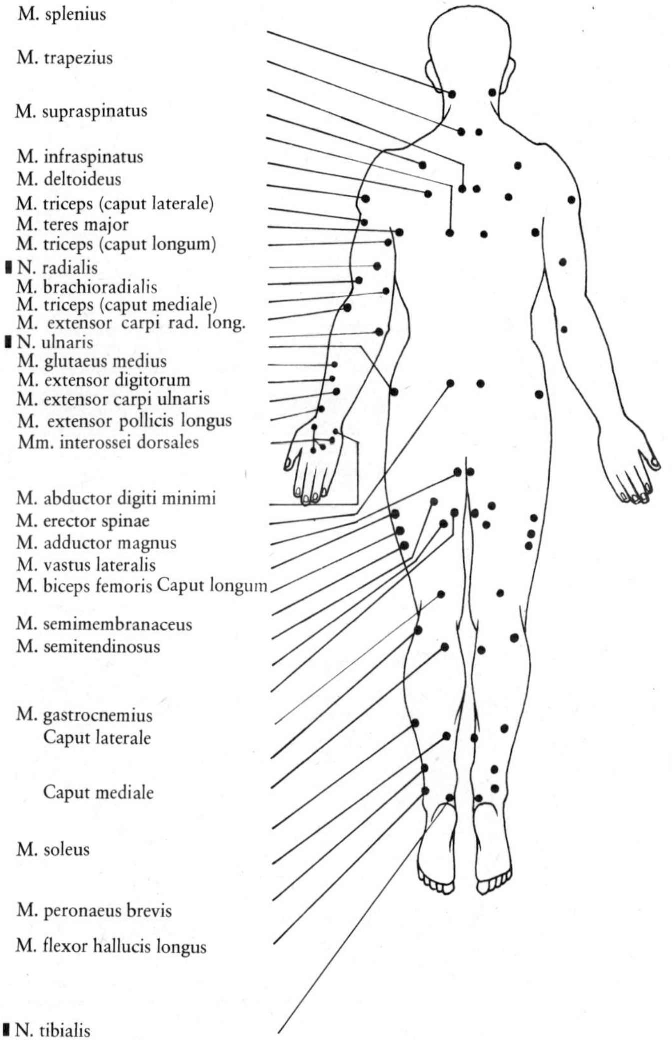

M. splenius

M. trapezius

M. supraspinatus

M. infraspinatus
M. deltoideus
M. triceps (caput laterale)
M. teres major
M. triceps (caput longum)
▮ N. radialis
M. brachioradialis
M. triceps (caput mediale)
M. extensor carpi rad. long.
▮ N. ulnaris
M. glutaeus medius
M. extensor digitorum
M. extensor carpi ulnaris
M. extensor pollicis longus
Mm. interossei dorsales

M. abductor digiti minimi
M. erector spinae
M. adductor magnus
M. vastus lateralis
M. biceps femoris Caput longum

M. semimembranaceus
M. semitendinosus

M. gastrocnemius
  Caput laterale

  Caput mediale

M. soleus

M. peronaeus brevis

M. flexor hallucis longus

▮ N. tibialis

FIG. 83.—Points of stimulation of important muscles and nerves, (▮): posterior view.

197

Table of Clinically Significant Muscle-Stretch Reflexes

Term	Effect	Nerve	Root
Biceps reflex	Arm flexion	Musculocutaneous N.	C5–C6
Brachioradialis reflex	Arm flexion	Radial N.	C5–C6
Triceps reflex	Arm extension	Radial N.	C6–C8
Pronator reflex	Pronation	Median N.	C6–C7
Pectoralis reflex	Arm adduction	Lat. pectoral N.	C5–C8
Adductor reflex	Leg adduction	Obturator N.	L2–L4
Quadriceps reflex	Knee-extension	Femoral N.	L2–L4
Internal hamstring reflex	Knee-flexion	Sciatic N.	S1
External hamstring reflex	Knee-flexion	Sciatic N.	S1–S2
Triceps surae reflex	Plantar flexion	Tibial N.	S1–S2
Posterior tibial reflex	Pronation	Tibial N.	L5
Superficial Reflexes			
Corneal reflex	Eyelid closure	Trigeminal and Facial N.	
Superficial abdominal reflexes	Movement of umbilicus		T7–T12
Cremaster reflex	Elevation of testicle	Genitofemoral N.	L1–L2
Anal reflex	Contraction of anal sphincter	Pudendal N.	S3–S5
Plantar reflex	Flexion of toes	Tibial N.	S1–S2
Mayer's sign	Thumb apposition and adduction	Median and Ulnar N.	C8–T1

Entrapment Neuropathies

Local mechanical compression (entrapment) of a specific peripheral nerve leading to its dysfunction occurs at predisposed, vulnerable anatomic sites.

Idiopathic facial nerve palsy: Compression within the facial canal (?). Signs: Unilateral paresis of facial musculature, platysma and stapedius muscle. Lesions proximal to geniculate ganglion lead to impairment of tear production (involvement of greater superficial petrosal nerve); more distal lesions within the canal to impairment of taste (chorda tympani).

Thoracic outlet syndrome: Lower brachial plexus irritation (C8–T1) and intermittent ischemia of the arm are observed by encroachment of bony, fascial and muscular structures on the neurovascular bundle located in the thoracic outlet. (Adson maneuver: Arm abduction obliterates radial pulse). Cervical rib?

Long thoracic nerve palsy: Develops in manual laborers after carrying heavy loads and is seen in combination with winging of the scapula.

Suprascapular nerve entrapment: Compression at suprascapular foramen leads to shoulder pain, and weakness of abduction and external rotation of the arm.

Posterior interosseus nerve syndrome: Inability to extend the digits at the metacarpophalangeal joints due to involvement of posterior interosseus nerve (motor branch of radial nerve) as it enters the supinator muscle. M. triceps and m. extensor carpi radialis and sensation are spared.

Ulnar nerve entrapment at the elbow: Entrapment of the ulnar nerve at the ulnar groove.

Pronator teres syndrome: Entrapment of the median nerve at the level of pronator teres muscle producing pain and paresthesias of the hand.

Carpal tunnel syndrome: Entrapment of the median nerve in the carpal tunnel of the hand (beneath the transverse carpal ligament) leads to numbness and paresthesias of the thumb, index and middle fingers (bothersome at night), followed by weakness and atrophy of the thenar muscles. Delayed sensory latency across the wrist.

Ilioinguinal syndrome: Trauma, scar tissue, surgical procedures can irritate the iliolinguinal nerve, leading to groin pain and altered sensation in the crural area.

Meralgia paresthetica: see page 93

Tarsal tunnel syndrome: Compresssion of posterior tibial nerve along the medial malleolus of the ankle leading to painful dysesthesias and intrinsic foot weakness.

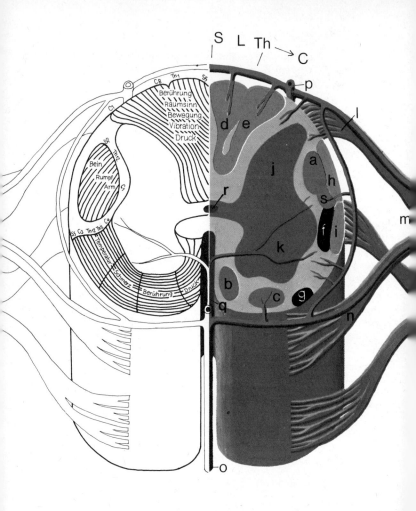

Fig. 84.—Topographic localization of the major tracts of the spinal cord according to Foerster. Berührung = touch, Bewegung = position, Druck = pressure, Bein = lower limb, Rumpf = trunk, Arm = upper limb. Temperatur = temperature, Schmerz = pain.

INCIDENCE OF THE MOST IMPORTANT NEUROLOGIC DISEASES
(Adapted from widespread literature sources; many figures have been estimated. Regional differences; some figures (*) from autopsy material.)

	Cases		Population
Cerebrovascular disease	1		7*
Ischemic infarcts	1		9
Intracerebral hematoma	1		14*
Cerebral emboli	1		50
Aneurysms	1		100*
Brain tumors	1		100*
Neuroepithelial tumors		ca. 50%	
Ecto- and mesodermal tumors		ca. 35%	
Cerebral metastases and other		ca. 25%	
Spinal cord tumors	1		2000
Neurofibroma		ca. 30%	
Meningioma		ca. 30%	
Neuroepithelial tumors		ca. 25%	
Spinal cord vascular lesions	1		150
Parkinsonian syndrome	1		200
Epilepsy	1		200
Occasional seizures	1		20
Disseminated encephalomyelitis	1		2000
Huntington's chorea	1		20,000
Friedreich's ataxia	1		25,000
Wilson's disease	1		20,000
Syringomyelia	1		10,000
Motor neuron disease	1		1000
Muscular dystrophies	1		4000
Myotonic dystrophy	1		20,000
Myasthenia gravis	1		30,000

Neurologic Disorders of Autosomal Dominant Inheritance
(adapted from P.E. Becker and G. Koch, 1966)

Pelizaeus-Merzbacher's disease — adult onset
Tuberous sclerosis
von Recklinghausen's neurofibromatosis
Familial gliomatosis cerebri
von Hippel-Lindau disease, cerebelloretinal angiomatosis
Sturge-Weber disease — with incomplete penetrance
Dystonia musculorum deformans
Progressive myoclonus epilepsy
Huntington's chorea
Parkinson's disease, rare type
Familial essential tremor
Wilson's disease (hepatolenticular degeneration)
Creutzfeldt-Jakob disease, occasionally familial
Hereditary areflexic dystasia (Roussy-Lévy syndrome)
Spastic paraplegia and distal muscle wasting (Troyer syndrome)
Hereditary spastic ataxia (Marie)
Olivopontocerebellar atrophy (Menzel)
Marinesco-Sjögren syndrome
Dyssynergia cerebellaris myoclonica (Ramsay-Hunt disease)
Hereditary spastic paraplegia
Familial amyotrophic lateral sclerosis
Scapuloperoneal muscular atrophy
Peroneal muscular atrophy (Charcot-Marie-Tooth disease)
Narcolepsy
Alzheimer's disease
Pick's disease
Facioscapulohumeral muscular dystrophy
Dystrophia myotonica
Myotonia congenita (Thomsen)
Distal muscular dystrophy (Welander)
Oculopharyngeal muscular dystrophy
Central-core disease
Nemaline myopathy
Centronuclear (myotubular) myopathy

Neurologic Disorders of Autosomal Recessive Inheritance

(adapted from P.E. Becker and G. Koch, 1966)

Metachromatic leukodystrophy—infantile and adult forms
Pelizaeus-Merzbacher's disease—infantile form
Globoid cell leukodystrophy (Krabbe)
Adrenoleukodystrophy, x-linked recessive
Alexander's disease
Famililal corticomeningeal angiomatosis (Divry-van Bogaert)
Ataxia telangiectasia (Louis-Bar syndrome)
Klippel-Trenaunay-Weber syndrome
Dystonia musculorum deformans
Progressive myoclonus epilepsy with Lafora inclusion bodies
Idiopathic basal ganglia calcification (Fahr's disease)
Friedreich's ataxia
Retinitis pigmentosa
Marinesco-Sjögren syndrome (spinocerebellar ataxia associated with congenital cataract and oligophrenia)
Dyssynergia cerebellaris myoclonica (Ramsay-Hunt)
A-beta-lipoproteinemia (Bassen-Kornzweig)
Hartnup's disease (amino-aciduria with cerebellar ataxia and a pellagra-like rash)
Heredopathia atactica polineuritiformis (Refsum's disease)
Familial spastic paraplegia
Congenital insensitivity to pain
Infantile spinal muscular atrophy (Werdnig-Hoffmann)
Juvenile spinal muscular atrophy (Kugelberg-Welander)
Hypertrophic neuropathy (Dejerine-Sottas)
X-linked recessive muscular dystrophies, Duchenne type and Becker-Kiener type

HEREDITARY METABOLIC DISEASES OF THE NERVOUS SYSTEM

All these disturbances eventually lead to marked intellectual deterioration (dementia), seizures [in those marked A] and spasticity [in those marked S]). Specific features listed.

Disease	Enzyme Defect	Syndrome
Carbohydrate metabolism		
Pompe's disease	α-1,4 glucosidase	
Galactosemia	Galactose 1-phosphate Uridyl transferase	
Fructose intolerance	Fructose-1 phosphate aldolase	
Mucolipidoses (gargoyl like features)	Thermolabile β-galactosidase (?)	
Mannosidase	α-mannosidase	
Fucosidase	α-L-fucosidase	S
Amino acid metabolism		
Phenylketonuria	Phenylalanine-hydroxylase	S
Histidinemia	Histidase	
Maple syrup urine disease	Branched chain alpha keto acid decarboxylase	A
Hypervalinemia	Valine transaminase	
Hyperglycinemia	3 types	A
Homocystinuria	Cystathionine synthetase	
Tyrosinemia	*p*-hydroxyphenyl pyruvic acid oxidase	
Urea cycle		
Citrullinemia	Argininosuccinate synthetase	A
Lipid metabolism		
GM$_1$-gangliosidosis	B-galactosidase	A
GM$_2$-gangliosidosis (Tay-Sachs' disease)	Hexosaminidase A	S, cherry red macula, A
Gaucher's disease	β-glucosidase	A, S
Globoid leukodystrophy (Krabbe's disease)	β-galactosidase	A, S, peripheral neuropathy

Metachromatic leukodystrophy	Arylsulfatase A	S, peripheral neuropathy
Fabry's disease	Ceramide trihexosidase	Vascular accidents, kidney failure, reddish purple skin rash
Refsum's disease	Phytanic acid-α-hydroxylase	Ataxia, retinitis pigmentosa, polyneuropathy
Niemann-Pick's disease	Sphingomyelinase	

(After Kanig, K., *Einf. i.d. allgemeine und klinische Neurochemie*, G. Fischer, Stuttgart, 1973.)

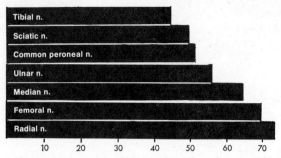

Fig. 85.—Normal values of motor nerve conduction velocity of clinically important peripheral nerves.

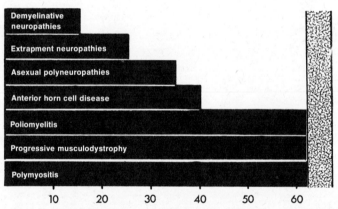

Fig. 86.—Motor nerve conduction velocities (m/sec) and alterations in selective neuromuscular disorders. (After Schadè: Einführung in die Neurologie 2 Aufl., G. Fischer Verlag, Stuttgart 1975.)

206

References

Books

Baker A. B. (Ed.): Clinical Neurology, Hoeber-Harper, New York 1965

Bodechtel G. (Ed.): Differentialdiagnose neurologischer Krankheitsbilder, 2nd edition, Thieme, Stuttgart 1974

Gänshirt H. (Ed.): Der Hirnkreislauf, Thieme, Stuttgart 1972

Haymaker W.: Bing's local diagnosis in neurological diseases, Mosby Co., St. Louis 1969

Heyck H., G. Laudahn: Die progressis-dystrophischen Myopathien, Springer, Berlin etc. 1969

Hopf H. C., A. Struppler: Elektromyographie, Thieme, Stuttgart 1974

Janzen R.: Elemente der Neurologie, Springer, Berlin 1969

Janz D.: Die Epilepsien, Thieme, Stuttgart 1969

Kugler J.: Die Elektroenzaphalographie in Klinik und Praxis, Thieme, Stuttgart 1966, 2nd edition

Mumenthaler M., H. Schliack: Läsionen peripherer Nerven, 2nd edition, Thieme, Stuttgart

Neundörfer B.: Differentialtypologie der Polyneuritiden, Springer 1973

Peters G.: Klinische Neuropathologie, 2nd edition, Thieme, Stuttgart 1970

Schaltenbrand G.: Allgemeine Neurologie, Thieme, Stuttgart 1969

Scheid W. (Ed.): Lehrbuch der Neurologie, Thieme, Stuttgart, 4th edition

Vinken P. J., G. W. Bruyn: Handbook of Clinical Neurology, North Holland Publishing Co. 1969

Zülch K.: Die Hirngeschwülste in biologischer und morphologischer Darstellung. J. A. Barth, Leipzig 1956

These books contain numerous references for further reading.

Journals

Aktuelle Neurologie (Thieme, Stuttgart). Brain (London). Fortschritte der Neurologie, Psychiatrie und ihrer Grenzgebiete (Thieme, St.). J. Neurology, Neurosurgery, Psychiatry (London). Nervenarzt (Springer, Berlin). Neurology (Minneapolis). Revue Neurologique (Paris). Zeitschrift f.

Neurologie (Springer, Berlin)

Zentralblatt f. d. ges. Neurologie und Psychiatrie (Springer, B.).

These journals provide an up-to-date review of the world literature.

Index of Neurologic Symptomatology and Syndromes

A

Abscess, cerebral, 22, 158, 182
Acalculia, 36, 37, 137, 166
Acoustic neuroma, 77, 129
Acromegaly, 173
Adenoma, basophilic pituitary,
174, 175
chromophobe, 174, 175
Adversive seizures, 28, 29
Agraphia, 36, 37, 137, 166
Ahylognosia, 36
Akinesia, 27, 134
Alexia, 36, 37, 137, 166
Alzheimer's disease, 179
Amaurosis fugax, 71
Amimia, 131, 135
Amnesia, retrograde, 161
Amorphognosia, 36
Amusia, 36, 166
Amytrophy, neuralgic, 68
Anemia, 189
Aneurysm, 43, 71, 73, 142, 186
Anosmia, 69, 166
Anosognosia, 39, 166
Anterior horn syndrome, 6, 47, 100
Anticoagulation, hemorrhage, 143,
165
Apallic syndrome, 163
Aphasia, 3, 7, 134, 137, 159, 166,
179, 189
motor, 37, 166
sensory, 36, 37, 189
Apraxia, 137, 166, 189
Arachnoiditis, 121
optico-chiasmatic, 71
Areflexia, 11, 69, 107, 111, 117
Argyll Robertson pupil, 153, 155
Arnold-Chiari syndrome, 121
Arteriovenous malformation, 43,
113, 127, 143, 172
Astereognosis, 36
Astrocytoma, 171, 172
Asynergia, 25, 127

Ataxia, 25, 77, 107, 117, 119, 153,
157, 205,
frontal, 166
lateral cerebellar tracts, 25, 107
Athetosis, 27, 133
Atonia, muscular, 11
Aura, 29, 166, 183
Automatisms, 17
Autonomic zones, 13, 67
Autotopagnosia, 37
Avellis's syndrome, 125
Axonotmesis, 12, 13, 15, 67
Azotemia, 189

B

Babinski's sign, 16, 33, 46, 107,
113, 133, 137, 163
Babinski-Nageotte's syndrome, 125
Bannwarth's syndrome, 75
Behçet's disease, 117, 147, 157
Bell's palsy, 75
Benedikt's syndrome, 125
Bing-Horton's syndrome, 189
Bladder, automatic, 19, 109
denervated, 96
function, disturbances, 16, 17,
19, 96, 107, 109, 119, 166
Blindness, 71, 153, 189
Blood pressure, raised, 139, 143,
189, 191
Bourneville's disease, 177
Brachial plexus palsy, 4, 8, 89, 98
Brain stem contusion, 161
Brissaud's syndrome, 125
Brown-Sèquard's syndrome, 4, 5,
19, 101
Bulbar palsy, 63, 79, 105

C

C7 syndrome, 4, 89, 192
Café au lait patches, 52
Carpal tunnel syndrome, 85

Cataract, 61
Cauda equina syndrome, 19, 115
Central core myopathy, 58, 59, 64
Cerebellar disorders 25, 127
Cerebellopontine angle tumors, 41,
  75, 128, 129
Cerebral death, 35
Céstan-Chenais' syndrome, 125
Cheiralgia paresthetica, 85
Chiray-Foix-Nicolesco's syndrome,
  125
Cholesteatoma, 147
Chondroma, 129
Chorea, 27, 133, 201
Choriomeningitis, lymphocytic, 147
Choroid plexus papilloma, 123, 173
Chronaxy, 9
Citrullinemia, 204
Claude's syndrome, 125
Claudication, intermittent spinal,
  109
Clivus syndrome, 73
Clubfoot, 95
Cogwheel phenomenon, 11, 131
Commotio cerebri, 161
Conduction velocity, of motor
  nerves, 206
Contusio cerebri, 160, 161
  brain stem, 57
Coordination, disturbances, 25
Craniopharyngioma, 174, 175
Crisis, cholinergic, 63
  myasthenic, 63
CSF, high pressure, 21
  high protein level, 23, 149, 169
  low pressure, 21
  occlusion of passages, 121
Cushing's syndrome, 59

D

Dandy-Walker syndrome, 121
Decerebration, 33, 35, 121, 163,
  179
Decubitus ulceration, 18, 19
Degeneration, hepatolenticular, 135
  reaction of (RD), 9, 91, 111

Dejerine-Sottas' disease, 109
Dementia, senile, 179
Dermatomyositis, 59
Diabetes, insipidus, 157
  mellitus, 52, 68, 137, 173, 189
Diathesis, hemorrhagic, 142
Disk prolapse, lateral, 90
  medial, 115
Dissociated sensory loss, 3
Dopamine, 131
Double vision, 35, 61, 73, 123,
  129, 157
Dream state, 166, 183
Dressing apraxia, 39, 129, 166
Dysarthria, 107, 135, 155
Dysmetria, 25

E

Edema, cerebral, 45, 139, 158,
  163, 167, 189
Embolism, cerebral, 137, 201
Encephalitis, bacterial, 159
  central European, 146, 159
  herpes, 149, 159
  lethargica, 131, 159
  postvaccination, 159
Encephalomyelitis, disseminated,
  22, 23, 119, 201
Enophthalmos, 88, 89, 111
Entrapment neuropathies, 199
Ependymitis, 121
Ependymoma, 112, 127, 129, 171,
  172
Epilepsy, early traumatic, 161, 181
  grand mal, 29, 180, 184
  impulsive petit mal, 29, 180, 183
  late traumatic, 163, 181
Erythrocytophages, 23, 145
Erythroprosopalgia, 189
Exanthem, 103
Extensor spasms, 33, 35, 121, 163,
  165

F

Fabry's disease, 205
Facial neuralgia, 188

palsy, 75, 119, 129, 157, 161, 199
Falx meningioma, 168, 169
Fever, 149, 157, 159, 161, 165
Finger agnosia, 36, 37, 166
Flapping tremor, 52
Flask sign, 85
Foot, club, 95
   Friedreich's, 105, 107
   talipes equinus, 18
Foramen, jugular, 79
   Luschka, 20, 120
   Magendie, 20, 120
   Monro, 20,21
Foster Kennedy's syndrome, 71
Foville's syndrome, 71, 125
Friedreich's ataxia, 101, 107, 201
   foot, 105, 107
Froment's sign, 87
Fructose intolerance, 204
Fucosidase, 204

G

Gait, stepping, 95
   waddling, 55
Galactosemia, 204
Gangliosidosis, 204
Gargoylism, 204
Gasperini's syndrome, 125
Gaucher's disease, 204
Generalized changes (EEG), 31, 35
   neurofibromatosis (von
      Recklinghausen), 52, 53, 176,
      177
Geographic skull, 41
German measles, 147
Gerstmann's syndrome, 37
Giant-cell arteritis (Horton), 137,
   189
Glioblastoma, 43, 139, 170
Glioma, 43, 111, 171
Gordon's knee sign, 133
   sign, 33
Grand mal seizure, 29, 180, 184
Granuloma, 131, 153, 157
Grasp reflex, 32, 33, 143, 166
Guillain-Barré syndrome, 23
Guillain-Garcin syndrome, 73

210

H

Hallucinations, 166
Hand, 111
   claw, 83, 87
   oath, 85
Hemangioma, 113
Hematoma, cerebral (hemorrhage),
   142, 143, 201
   epidural, 45, 115, 164
   intracranial, 41, 43, 142
   subdural, 45, 162, 165, 190
Hemianopia, bitemporal, 70, 71
   contralateral (homonymous), 38,
      70, 71, 137, 166
Hemiballismus, 27, 135
Hemihypesthesia, 4, 5, 46, 125,
   137, 166
Hemiparesis, 7, 46, 137, 143, 166
Hemiplegia alternans, 73, 75, 123,
   125
Hemisomatagnosia, 39
Hemisphere, dominant, 37, 166
   nondominant, 38, 39, 166
Hemophilia, 93
Hemosiderin phagocytes, 23, 145
Heredoataxia, 106, 211
Herpes simplex, 53, 149, 159
   zoster, 101, 103, 149
Heubner's syphilitic endarteritis,
   153
Histidinemia, 204
Homocystinuria, 204
Horner's syndrome, 88, 89, 111,
   123
Horton's syndrome, 189
Hydrocephalus, 120, 121, 157, 179
Hydrophobia, 159
Hyperacusis, 77
Hyperglycinemia, 204
Hyperkalemia (hypo-), 65
Hyperkinesia, 27, 133
Hypermetria, 25
Hyperpathia, 5
Hyperpyrexia, malignant, 65
Hyperreflexia, 11
Hypertension, 137, 142, 145
Hyperthyroidism, 59

Hypervalinemia, 204
Hypesthesia, 3, 69, 119
Hypoglycemia, 189
Hypokalemia, 189
Hyporeflexia, 11
Hypotonia, muscle, 11, 68, 107,
    153, 187

I

Idiopathic facial nerve palsy, 199
Impulsive petit mal, 29, 180, 183
Infarct, ischemic, 201
Injection damage, 95
Intention tremor, 25, 119
Intracranial hypertension, 21, 34,
    35, 47, 122, 159, 167

J

Jacksonian attack, 29, 155, 166
    sensory, 166
Jackson's syndrome, 79, 125
Jacod's syndrome, 73

K

Kayser-Fleischer corneal rings, 133
Krabbe's disease, 191

L

L5 syndrome, 8, 91, 184
Lambert-Eaton syndrome, 63
Lasègue's sign, 48, 91
Lead poisoning, 68
Leukodystrophies, 67, 204
Louis-Bar's syndrome, 52
Lumbar plexus lesion, 97
Lupus erythematosus, 117, 157
Lyssa fever, 159

M

Mannosidase, 204
Maple syrup urine disease, 204
Marchand-Waterhouse syndrome,
    151

Mask facies, 60, 61, 63, 131
McArdle's syndrome, 65
Measles, 147
    German, 147
Medullary sheath degeneration,
    118
Medulloblastoma, 127, 129
Megalographia, 25, 107
Melkersson-Rosenthal's syndrome,
    75, 147
Meniére's disease, 77
Meningioma, 34, 41, 43, 112, 127,
    167, 172, 201
    clivus, 128
    convexity, 168, 169
    falx, 168, 169
    olfactory groove, 71, 169
    sphenoid wing, 169
    tuberculum sellae, 71, 169
Meningitis, carcinomatous, 148
    lymphocytic, 22, 23, 146
    purulent, 22, 23, 146
    syphilitic, 153
    tuberculous, 23, 154, 157
Meningoencephalopathy, 153
Meralgia paresthetica, 93
Metabolic diseases, 204, 205
Metabolism, disturbances of, 52
Metastases, 5, 113, 172, 173, 190
Micrographia, 131
Midbrain syndrome, 35, 47, 143,
    162, 165
Migraine, 187, 190
Millard-Gubler's syndrome, 75, 125
Miosis, 88, 89, 111
Mononucleosis, infectious, 147
Monro-Kellie doctrine, 35
Motor nerve conduction velocity,
    206
Multiple sclerosis, 22, 71, 73, 118
Mumps, 147
Muscle atrophy, 9, 97
    neural, 14, 69
    spinal, 14, 87, 104
Muscle dystrophy, 54, 64, 201
Muscle stretch reflexes, 198
Myasthenia gravis, 7, 62, 201
Mycosis, 146, 149

Mydriasis, 73
Myelitis, trauma, 101, 117
Myelomalacia, angiodysgenetic, 107
Myelopathy, vascular, 109
Myoglobinuria, 65
Myopathies, congenital, 59, 64
  functional, 65
Myositis, 56, 59
Myositis ossificans, 163
Myotonia congenita (Thomsen), 60, 61
Myotonia, dystrophica, 61, 201

N

Narcolepsy, 191
Neck stiffness, 145, 149, 157
Neglect, 39, 139, 166
Nemaline myopathy, 59, 64
Nerve, abducent, 72, 73, 98, 125, 129, 161
  axillary, 83, 98
  dorsal scapular, 81
  facial, 76, 119, 129, 157
  femoral, 4, 93, 98
  glossopharyngeal, 79
  lateral femoral cutaneous, 93
  long thoracic, 81, 98
  median, 3, 12, 84, 85, 98
  musculocutaneous, 83, 98
  obturator, 92
  oculomotor, 72, 98, 161
  suprascapular, 81
  tibial, 12, 95, 98
  trochlear, 73, 98, 161
  ulnar, 3, 12, 86, 98
Neuralgia, facial, 188
Neurologic disorders, incidence 201
  inheritance, 202, 203
Neuroma, 41, 112
Neuromyotonia, 65
Neurapraxia, 12, 13, 15
Neuropathies, entrapment, 199, 152
Neurosyphilis, 22, 152

Nickerson-Kveim reaction, 157
Niemann-Pick's disease, 205
Nothnagel's syndrome, 125
Nystagmus, 75, 119, 122, 184
  rotatory, 77

O

Oligodendroglioma, 41, 170, 171
Opisthotonos, 149
Oppenheim's sign, 33
Optic atrophy, 71, 119, 153, 166
Oral petit mal, 29
Orientation, disturbance of spatial, 39, 139, 166

P

Pain, lancinating, 49, 117
Palsy, idiopathic facial nerve, 199
  long, thoracic nerve, 199
Pancoast's tumor, 89
Papilledema, 71
Paraglioma, 171
Paralysis, 7, 69
  Lissauer's, 153
  progressive, 23, 155
Paraphasia, 37
Paraplegia, spastic, 18
  transverse myelopathy, 3, 7, 16, 47, 113, 114, 115, 117, 119
Parasites, 23, 149
Paresthesias, 3, 13, 69, 107, 119
Parinaud's syndrome, 125
Parkinsonian syndrome, 27, 131, 134, 159, 201
Pellagra, 52
Periarteritis nodosa, 68, 117, 157
Personality change, epileptic, 185
Petit mal, 29, 31
  pyknoleptic, 180, 183
Phakomatoses, 177
Phenylketonuria, 52, 204
Pheochromocytoma, 189
Photophobia, 159
Pick's disease, 179
Pill rolling 131

Pinealoma, 173
Pituitary adenomas, 175
Pleocytosis, 23, 119, 145, 149
Poliomyelitis, anterior, 23, 101, 103
Polycythemia, 189
Polymyositis, 56, 59
Polyneuritis, 3, 8, 25, 52, 68, 99, 157, 205
Polyneuropathy (Dejerine-Sottas), 69
Pompe's disease, 204
Porphyria, 52, 69
Precocious puberty, 173
Predilection paralysis, 9, 139
Pressure sella, 34, 35, 41, 167, 190
Primitive phenomena, 33, 145, 163
Propulsion, 131
Propulsive petit mal, 180
Psoas hematoma, 93
Ptosis, 73, 88, 89, 111, 123
Pudendal plexus lesion, 97
Pupil, dilatation, 165
Pyknolepsy, 180, 183
Pyramidal tract signs, 11, 33, 105, 107, 111, 119, 122, 125, 131, 137, 157, 163, 165, 166

Q

Quadrantic hemianopia, 71, 167
Queckenstedt's sign, 21, 101, 113

R

Rachischisis, 121
Radial palsy, 68, 82
Raymond-Céstan syndrome, 125
Reflexes, muscle stretch, 198
Refsum's disease, 52, 205
Resorcinol myopathy, 59
Respiratory paralysis, 63, 69, 103
Retinocerebellar angiomatosis, 177
Rhabdomyolysis, 65
Right-left disturbance, 36, 37, 166
Rigidity, 11, 131, 134
Rossolimo's sign, 17
Roussy-Lévy syndrome, 107

S

S1 syndrome, 91, 192
Salaam spasms (propulsive petit mal), 29, 180, 183, 184
Saliva, excess, 77, 131
Sarcoidosis, 75, 147, 157
Sayk preparation, 22
Scapula, winged, 57
Schmidt's syndrome, 125
Scholz's disease, 204
Scoliosis, 103
Seizures, focal 167, 182, 183
    grand mal, 29, 180, 184
    jacksonian, 29, 155, 166
    myoclonic-astatic, 29, 180
    petit mal, 29, 31
    psychomotor, 180, 183
    symptomatic, 185
Sensation, disturbances of, 3, 5
Serratus anterior, paralysis of, 81
Siebenmann's syndrome, 79
Snout reaction, 33, 143, 163
Spasticity, 11, 105, 107, 109, 111, 113, 115, 117, 119, 127, 139, 163, 204
Spastic torticollis, 27, 133
Speech, scanning, 119
    slurred, 25
Spikes and waves (SW), 31
Spina bifida, 121
Spinal paralysis, spastic, 104
Spongioblastoma, 123, 171
Spontaneous fracture, 153
Status demyelinatus, 133
    epilepticus, 184
    marmoratus, 133
Stiff-man syndrome, 65
Sturge-Weber's disease, 52, 177
Subarachnoid hemorrhage, 144, 160, 191
Subscapular nerve entrapment, 199
Supinator canal syndrome, 83
Suture diastasis, 41
Syndrome, angular, 141
    anterior cerebral artery, 137, 141
    apallic, 163

213

anterior choroidal artery, 141
anterior parietal artery, 141
anterior temporal artery, 141
carpal tunnel, 199
great radicular artery of
  Adamkiewicz, 109
ilioinguinal, 199
internal carotid artery, 139, 141
meningitic, 22, 23, 147
middle cerebral artery, 137, 141
occipital artery, 123
posterior cerebral artery, 137,
  141
posterior cranial fossa, 47, 126,
  128
posterior interosseus nerve, 199
posterior spinal artery, 100, 108
preolandic artery, 141
pronator teres, 199
spinocerebellar, 107
superior orbital fissure, 73
tarsal tunnel, 199
thoracic outlet, 199
Syringobulbia, 111
Syringomyelia, 3, 19, 88, 101, 110

T

Tabes dorsalis, 25, 69, 116, 153
Tapia's syndrome, 125
Tetra/hemiparesis, 7, 109, 123
Tetraspasticity, 128
Thalamus, disturbances, 5
Tongue biting, 28, 29, 181
Torsion dystonia, 27, 133
Toxoplasmosis, 146
Trauma, craniocerebral, 161
Tremor, 27, 131, 133
Trendelenburg's sign, 55

Trigeminal neuralgia, 188
Trigger zones, 75, 188
Trömner's sign, 17
Tuberculosis, CNS, 23, 154, 157
Tuberose sclerosis, 52, 71, 177
Tumor, cerebral, 22, 23, 34, 35,
  127, 167, 187, 190
  psychosis, 171
  spinal, 3, 19, 22, 101, 111
  suprasellar, 175
Tyrosinose, 191

U

Uncinate fit, 71, 166

V

Vernet's syndrome, 79, 125
Vestibular (acoustic) neuroma, 77,
  129
Virus meningitis, 22, 146
Visual hallucinations, 166
  contralateral (homonymous), 162
Vomiting, 34, 35, 129, 145, 161,
  167, 187
von Hippel-Lindau' disease, 52,
  127, 177
von Recklinghausen's disease, 53,
  176, 177

W

Wallenberg's syndrome, 125, 127
Weber's syndrome, 73, 125
Wernicke-Mann type of
  hemiparesis, 9, 46, 139
Whiplash injury, cervical spine,
  115

214